What Doctors Don't Get to Study in Medical School

What Doctors Don't Get to Study in Medical School

BM Hegde
MD, FRCP, FRCPE, FRCPG, FRCPI, FACC, FAMS
Visiting Prof Cardiology, The Middlesex Hospital
Medical School, University of London
Affiliate Prof of Human Health, Northern Colorado University
Visiting Prof Indian Institute of Advanced Studies, Shimla
Retd. Vice Chancellor, MAHE University, Manipal.

Paras Medical Publisher
Solutions for Health Care Professionals

Anshan

What Doctors Don't Get to Study in
Medical School

First published in the UK by

ANSHAN LTD
In 2006

6 Newlands Road, Tunbridge Wells,
Kent. TN4 9AT. UK
Tel/Fax: +44 (0) 1892 557767
e-mail: info@anshan.co.uk
Web Site: www.anshan.co.uk

Published in arrangement with
Paras Medical Publisher, 5-1-475 First Floor
Putlibwoli, Hyderabad - 500 095, India.
E-mail: parasmedpub@hotmail.com

© BM Hegde

ISBN 10: 1 904 79884 5
ISBN 13: 978 1 904798 84 2

All rights reserved. No part of this publication may be reproduced, stored in a retrieval system, or transmitted in any form or by means, electronic, mechanical, photocopying, recording and/or otherwise, without the prior written permission of the publishers.

Note: This is not a conventional textbook and, as such, need not be depended on for examination purposes. Much of what is written here might not be known to conventional examiners. This is the bible for an inquisitive, dedicated, and an authentic doctor to get to know the truth behind the present day medical claptrap. This is not also an authentic pharmacopoeia for patients to follow. They must follow their treating doctors' advice. The author is not responsible for the readers not following the above suggestions and the consequences thereof. In view of the possibility of human error or advances in medical science neither the editor nor the publisher nor any other party who has been involved in the preparation or publication of this work warrants that the information contained herein is in every respect accurate or complete.

British Library Cataloguing in Publication Data
A catalogue record for this book is available from the British Library

To

My parents and teachers for their inspiration
My wife, daughters, son, sons-in-law and
my grandchildren for their support and love

FOREWORD

There are several compelling reasons why different groups among the millions of users and friends of Whole Person Healing (often misleadingly called by the US Government "Complementary and Alternative Medicine", CAM) should read this book. First, let me paraphrase Hippocrates (*who better on a book for medical students?*): "It is more important to know the author than the book that she/he has written". In the original it said: *"It is more important to know the person than the disease the person has."* That is still true.

I have known the author, Dr BM Hegde for less than a year, starting when both he and I spoke at a historic meeting in the great hall of the Indian National Science Academy (INSA) in October, 2004. This meeting, which I helped initiate, was convened by the Director General of the CSIR (Dr RA Mashelkar) and the President of INSA (Dr MS Valiathan). It was on a subject which could *never* have been allowed in the corresponding venue by the similar executives in any other country in the world. The focus was on the "Science of Traditional Healing." The conveners and I were speakers there, but I was most impressed by the content *and* the style of the talk by Dr Hegde. What was impressive in that context, as it is in this book, is that he spoke from the position of leadership in the hard-core western medicine world, and he spoke from his heart and head at the same time. He is a senior, learned practitioner and researcher, and administrator in that world of allopathic medicine. Hence what *he* says in constructive criticism of the world of current (allopathic) medical practice, carries weight which those outside the field, like myself, cannot aspire to. Moreover, what drew me to him was his forthright style: he called spades, "spades"; and gave the well-established figures on the failures of the high-tech medical world with gusto and authority.

Every foreword should inform the reader about what kind of audience would most benefit from this book. Although he says this cannot be a "textbook", clearly the author intends it for the students and graduates of the world of academic medicine (mainly allopathic). For them, I believe it *should be required reading*, but it will certainly be part of the *important* and formative reading we all do outside the requirements for a degree. Here, laid out concisely, are all the rather well-established potholes and pitfalls in current medical thinking and practice. The exceptional value of this work by Dr Hegde is that solid data have been clearly pulled out and catalogued from the literature and put into punchy, attention-getting form.

In his chapter on "Need-based education" his sound comments on philosophy, pedagogy, even examinations of various kinds, brings out his wisdom born of long experience as department head and Dean and Vice-Chancellor.

But Dr Hegde's work will have equal value to the vast numbers of practitioners of Whole Person Healing—acupuncturists, chiropractors, naturopaths, Reiki masters, electromagnetic device manufacturers, etc., etc. Why? Because they will see that the claims of much of high-tech medicine are riddled with doubt compared to the glossy advertising, and even papers, whether in NEJM, BMJ or in the local newspaper advertisements for Nexium or Viagra. His critiques of the absurd over-reliance on *technology* of dial-watching instead of pulse-taking, of the profound role of *money* instead of caring, are distorting the healing vector in deep and profound ways. His positive exposition of the role of rhythm and holism is an appropriate counterweight.

Let me comment on his *style* from the viewpoint of a physical-chemist-materials scientist. What I salute is his utilization of relevant data and facts, with little attention to explanations, mechanisms and theories. In this he follows the call of Aristotle, writing in Nicomachean Ethics:

"Nor again must we in all matters alike demand an explanation of the reason why things are what they are; in some cases it is enough if the fact that they are so satisfactorily established. This is the case with first principles; and the fact is the primary thing—it is a first principle."

Medical science has overrun its headlights—following the arcane parts of physics. It aims for explanation, theories, elegance, what it lacks in data. Instead of electron-micrographs, we see "cartoons" of alleged structures. After a headline says "New drug shows promise of cure for XYX" the demurrer phrase about side effects repeated ad nauseam is always in small print or well hidden. Dr Hegde reaches far and wide for data. The book is loaded with excellent and valuable references for all honest medical-scientists who seek to improve their fields instead of merely mining it to make a very good living.

The key ideas are often leaked out to the reader very effectively in the chapter headings and highlighted quotes at the beginning. For example, to introduce "Health Care Delivery" (in India) he opens with the quote,

"The thinking that doctors and hospitals are needed to keep a society healthy is plain rubbish."

This profound truth has many parents. No one has ever challenged it, but it is uniformly ignored. My Penn State colleague, and brilliant social philosopher, Ivan Illich, modern pioneer of this viewpoint, author of Medical *Nemesis* (1975), told many similar tales, and gave other data like those cited in this book, in **this** case by a leading medical professional with a plethora of data. Indeed, comparing the data between Illich and Hegde, one can see that in the 30 years between them, things have gotten even worse. Hegde correctly uses the pitiful state of US Healthcare as revealed in absolutely unchallenged data such as in the recent papers and books of Starfield and Angell to make his point that India should "not follow the footsteps of USA." I go much further. The USA healthcare system is a terminal patient in the "ICU". It is the existence theorem for the proof of the proposition that for-profit healthcare is an oxymoron. Profiting from the pain of others sounds intrinsically contradictory, as it has always been. The healing intention is an agapeic vector. India has the potential, using its own healing and social traditions, combined with its own hi-tech abilities to design a multi-level healthcare system, which distributes the benefits in a radically different *but sustainable* ratio than in the US model. Good primary care for all (free), modest secondary care for many (*partially* subsidized in order to retain the element of taking responsibility for one's own health), tertiary care for the few (largely out of pocket). Hegde's approaches are developed in depth in his chapter on the "Future Medicare System," which is wise counsel for all of us thinking about this unavoidable topic.

I salute the author also for not falling into the trap of fashionable pseudoscience, repeating the mantras or "halowords" like "quantum" and "consciousness" several times on the page. His short introduction to chaos theory is *relevant*; and intelligible. But he "stays on message": healing humans.

He introduces the place of, and the relevance and importance of, "CAM", which we have now made more accurate as "WPH", with interesting anecdotes, and references to India's own great healing tradition of Ayurveda—on which he has of course written elsewhere in depth.

I salute him also for dealing with the fundamentals of a *health* care not a disease management system, with "health expectancy" not life-expectancy. In a talk he gave in Washington in April 2005, Dr Hegde's critique of health screening were echoed in the plenary paper by the esteemed Dr Larry Dossey, who gave the latest statistics on the dangers of screening, and regular testing of populations.

Let me end this foreword with a comment on what is demonstrated by the author's **style**. First, his "catholicity" *and* his scholarship—he quotes equally from Sanskrit texts, and all the Greek and European *philosophers* and, of course, healers across 3000 years. But most importantly he does it with certain panache, a fearless and zesty style. *That* is the characteristic most missing in modern science and medicine today. I would say: Read this book to get a taste of the quality of "enthusiasm" (the etymology of "enthusiasm" links it to "en-theos", through God [the Spirit]) from a brilliant and committed author, if for no other reason!

University Park PA
August 5, 2005

Rustum Roy
Founding Director, Materials Research Laboratory
Evan Pugh Professor, Emeritus
Professor of Science, Technology, and Society, Emeritus
The Pennsylvania State University
Distinguished Visiting Professor in Materials
The Arizona State University
Visiting Professor of Medicine, Program in Integrative Medicine
The University of Arizona

ACKNOWLEDGEMENTS

I wish to thank all my teachers, friends, colleagues, secretaries, students, and patients for their help. My publishers, Paras Medical Publishers, have done a wonderful job. I must mention one name in particular of Mr Divyesh A Kothari, who has been instrumental in motivating me to write this book. He has been after me for a long time and I had no option but to oblige him. I must admit that it was pleasure working with him and his colleagues at Paras.

BM Hegde
"Manjunath" Pais Hills, Bejai
Mangalore-575 004, India.

CONTENTS

1. Introduction 1
2. Man and His Problems 5
3. Human Body's Intelligence 7
4. Societal Health Promotion 11
5. Health Care–Reaching the Unreached 17
6. Power of Prayer 23
7. The Art of Medicine 27
8. The Fine Art of Living 34
9. Doctors' Dilemma 39
10. Joys and Sorrows 42
11. Matter of the Mind 47
12. On Doctoring 52
13. Future Medicare System 59
14. Medical Philosophy 66
15. Primum Non Nocere (First, Do No Harm) 71
16. Primary Health Care 77
17. The Patient that Changed my Life 83
18. Medical Consultation 88
19. Medical Teleology 92
20. Limits of Science 97
21. Modern Medicine and Quantum Physics 102
22. Ultra-Science 108
23. Problems in the Evidence of Evidence-Based Medicine 113
24. Nanotechnology 116

25. Modern Medical Research-Time is Ripe for its Audit 120
26. Chaos – A New Science 125
27. Where is the Mind? Never Mind! 128
28. Euboxic Medicine 134
29. Evidence Based or Evidence Burdened Medicine? 139
30. Is Cancer a Disease? 144
31. Interventional Cardiology 149
32. Is Artificial Heart a Reality? 156
33. Life Expectancy Versus Health Expectancy 160
34. Mitral Valve Prolapse Syndrome 165
35. Ne Plus Ultra 168
36. Woman, Moon and Menstruation 173
37. Critical Care: More Things Not to Do 177
38. Antibiotic Crisis – A Time Bomb? 180
39. Needless Interventions in Medicine 183
40. Mothers, Babies, and Killer Diseases 188
41. Science and the Tower of Babel 191
42. Scientific Superstitions 194
43. Uncertainty is the only Certainty 199
44. Need-Based Medical Education 202
45. Health Care Delivery in India Today 211
46. Eye of the Beholder 217
47. Need for a Paradigm Shift in Medical Philosophy 222
48. Modern Medicine and Ancient Indian Wisdom 227
49. What is Yoga and What is not Yoga? 242
50. Health Scare System 246
51. Medical Education in India 252
52. How Might the Benefits of Ayurveda be Combined
    with Modern Medicine? 257
53. Holistic Lifestyle Changes for Wellness 262
54. Hormesis – One Man's Meat is another Man's Poison 270
Afterword 274

CHAPTER 1

Introduction

The title of the book needs an explanation. It is not that doctors deliberately neglect to study certain things in medical school that we need another book to tell them all about the *missing links*. Medical education needs drastic changes all over the world for doctors to be better equipped to deal with fellow human beings unfortunately suffering from illnesses, some real and many imaginary. The present education is disease oriented and not patient oriented. This must change first. Most of what we teach is based on statistical data that does not have a firm basis. Most of the data about illnesses, their causes, and their management could all be due to sheer chance or fluke, although we try to eliminate the possibility of fluke playing a part by applying statistical tests in research. In short, most of the science of medicine is not true science but statistical science.

Modern Medicine has been completely hijacked by technology and has been taken to the market place in the last couple of decades, resulting in medicine getting dehumanized and totally mechanized. The time tested doctor-patient relationship is at its nadir. Doctors are looked upon with suspicion by the lay man and the trust that they reposed in us is no longer there. Consumerism has come into the field in such a way that in the west, doctors practise defensive medicine more to save their own skin rather than to benefit the patient. This has resulted in untold misery and hardship to patients; in addition, modern medicine has become top heavy with technology and, consequently, is prohibitively expensive.

Recent studies in the West, both in the UK and the USA, have unequivocally shown that medical education from day one in the medical school is controlled by the money power of the multinational pharmaceutical giants and the technology manufacturers. Two recent editorials (in 2000 AD), one in *The Lancet* and another in *The New England Journal of Medicine* have shown how these operate stealthily without the students and, even most of the practising doctors, realizing the gravity of the problem. The modus operandi of these operators is revealed in an exhaustive editorial entitled *Looking the Gift Horse in the Mouth*, in a recent issue of the *Journal of American Medical Association*. To cap it, the editor who wrote the editorial mentioned above in the *NEJM*, Marcia Angell, who has been there for two decades as the editor-in-chief, after her husband, Relman, who was there for the previous two decades, resigned from the job after the management decided to change the editorial policy of not getting the editorials written by specialists with pharmaceutical company connections.

Marcia Angell has written an excellent book, *The Truth About Drug Companies-How they deceive us: What to do about it,* published by Random House, in which one gets an exhaustive account of the dealings going on behind the back of the custodians of human health. It is a sad commentary. As if that is not enough, another well researched book by a fellow American, John Abramson, *Overdo$ed America,* published by Harper Collins, is more revealing. This present book was planned way ahead of both those events because of my frustrations with the educational system in the medical schools, which I could not change despite the fact that I had occupied almost all important teaching positions. I failed miserably and got frustrated as, at every level, I had to meet with very stiff opposition for change. Those who keep in touch with medical literature know of my efforts in the last four decades.

While this could not be a textbook for the graduate students in medical colleges as they have to pass the conventional examinations based on the reductionist ideas that are taught, it will be a compelling companion for every medical doctor after passing the first MBBS examination and throughout his/her career, both during the clinical years in the college and later during medical practice forever. The book tries to give the reader an insight into the true realities in this field and also reveals the hidden flaws in the very basis of our understanding of the teaching and learning systems. I hope this achieves its goal of making doctors to *think*. Change comes only when one starts to think.

In the present information-loaded medical education, as in any other field of learning, the student does not get stimulated to think and be creative. This is not encouraged and the student who tries to do that gets left out of the mainstream and has the prospect of being a loser. No one wants to be a loser and so everyone catches up. After sometime, it becomes second nature, with the student getting inured to it. Doctors start believing in all that they are told and what they get to read. Most of what comes out in the plethora of biomedical journals is fake and doctored, but it is difficult to convince the readers about it. This book would try and cover those areas where there is a dense cloud of mist in our understanding of the very basis of medicine.

The human body is a dynamic system that is constantly being run by food and oxygen. All dynamic systems in this universe work as a whole and in tune with the environment. Hence, the human body works as a whole. Consequently, the human body has an inbuilt repair mechanism that works all the time to set things right when they go wrong. This repair mechanism works so well in this complicated machine that the body must have its own wisdom to find out the deviations as also its need for repair. There are well over one hundred thousand billion cells in the human system and all of them need to be in touch with one another to work smoothly and efficiently. Hence, the study of human physiology must, per force, understand the whole organism and its surroundings.

All dynamic systems in this universe follow the laws of holism and are governed by a new science, the science of CHAOS, which understands the basic working of the human body. Human body also follows different rhythms for its day-to-day activities. Most functions of the human body follow the *circadian rhythm,* where the changes take place approximately once in twenty-four hours. Some other functions follow the *ultradian rhythm* where changes occur many times in a day. Woman menstruates once in twenty-eight days, which is outside both the above rhythms. Menstruation is governed by another rhythm called *infradian rhythm.* All these three rhythms have their higher controls and the infradian rhythm is governed by the gravitational pull of the Moon.

Modern medicine was accepted by the European Universities as a science only in the twelfth century. Up until then it was considered to be sorcery, witchcraft, mumbo-jumbo and magic. It was around that time that medicine started following the natural sciences of physics, chemistry and biology. Medicine got lost in the then prevailing reductionist science of deterministic predictability. Medical scientists were also following the Cartesian model of reductionism. Although physics in the early twentieth century deviated from this concept and went headlong into the quantum field, medicine did not follow suit. It still got bogged down in reductionism. In the last fifty years, technology took charge of modern medicine in a big way and the science of reductionism became the firm foundation of medicine.

Human physiology is taught and understood in this background even today. Unfortunately, the human body does not follow the linear reductionist rules. This is where all our present problems in medicine arise. We study the organs of the body in isolation and plan our interventions, both drugs and surgical interventions, based on those wrong presumptions. This has resulted in a new class of problems for our patients, the iatrogenic (doctor induced) diseases, which have grown out of control now. It is reported that in one year in the United States of America, whose total population is around a quarter of India's population, more than 225,000 patients die because of wrong interventions and around 100,000 people meet their maker due to adverse drug reactions not known to the establishment. More than thirty million people suffer chronic illnesses due to doctors' interventions. All this and more could be avoided if we try and change our thinking in this field from that of reductionism to that of holism. This book attempts to unravel the mystery of human physiology in that setting using the holistic science of Chaos and fractals.

FURTHER READING

- Editorial. Drug Company Influence on Medical Education in the US. *Lancet.* 2000; 356:781.
- Angell M. Is Academic Medicine for Sale? *New Engl J Med.* 2000; 342: 1516–1518.
- Editorial. Looking the gift horse in the mouth. *JAMA* 2000; April issue.
- Angell M. *The Truth About Drug Companies*. 2004. Random House, New York.
- Abramson J. *Overdo$ed America*. 2004. Harper Collins, New York.

CHAPTER 2

Man and His Problems

Man has been evolving and living on this planet for well over 9,00,000 years in about 50,000 generations. How did we survive this long on this planet? The basic secret of our long survival is the inherent "**WISDOM OF THE HUMAN BODY.**" This is aided and abetted by our environment, which has an important say in this business. **"Contrary to popular belief, natural selection usually restrains evolution, which would otherwise happen at the mutation rate, by weeding out those mutated variants which would cope less well"** Even if the environments differed slightly than the present, successful living organisms would be totally different; dinosaurs would have survived and man would have been extinct instead!

Today, man, mesmerized by the reductionist scientific developments, including the advances in modern medicine, is led to believe that he could control all these with his technology, modern drugs and surgical feats. In addition, recently tall claims of successes in genetic engineering and also cloning have raised human hopes to the skies. Serious audit, of course, did not give credence to this belief. Illnesses and death without any drastic change still plague man even today just as in the last several centuries. Even the claims of **"epidemic rise and subsequent fall of degenerative diseases has been shown to be fallacious."** The graph of cancer death has not shown a tendency to come down although we have seen some improvements in certain childhood cancers. Hi-tech modern medicine is far from winning the war against cancer.

Modern medicine has been there with all its gadgets for the last 4–5 decades, but man survived here long before that without any of those gimmicks. **"Modern medicine, for all its breathtaking advances, seems**

to be slightly off balance like the Tower of Pisa," was the opinion of Prince Charles, the heir to the British throne. The one system of holistic health management that existed since the dawn of man's history is the Indian system of ***Ayurveda (the science of life).*** There are now enough evidences to say that this was the mother of all systems of medicine. A great Greek writer, E Pococke, in his celebrated book, **India in Greece**, has given evidence that Greek civilization was originally taken from India by Indians who migrated to Greece!

The advantage of this system is that it aids and abets ***Nature*** to keep man healthy and happy, if followed properly. It caters to the body, mind, and also the soul. The present WHO's definition of health takes into account all the three. The shortsighted modern reductionist scientific medicine looks at diseases from a narrow point of view. The latter would be beneficial in an emergency set up; but might even harm man in the long run. Antibiotic resistance is one such example. In the field of other advances, like genetic engineering, the omens are not that good, going by what we observe in the genetically modified plant kingdom!

Modern medicine is analogous to the fire fighting system. When the house is already on fire, with some parts of the house destroyed, the fire fighters try to quench the fire with water hoses. But in biology this kind of fire fighting results in the hose being short of the fire in many instances. Having realized the importance of holistic healing, many have now become interested in our ancient wisdom of Ayurveda that supplements the wisdom of the human body for survival. Indians in its land of birth have been lukewarm in their approach to Ayurveda, thanks to the colonial experience.

FURTHER READING

- Lakshmikantham. History of *Human Past—Children of Immortal Bliss*, 2002. Bharatiya Vidya Bhavan, Mumbai, India.
- Pococke E, *India In Greece*. 1832. Oxford University Press.

CHAPTER 3

Human Body's Intelligence

Man should have been extinct like the dinosaurs long ago if what we hear today about drugs, preventive screening of the apparently healthy population and technology keeping people alive on this planet were to be true. The latter were operational, at best, for little over half a century.

Many studies have been looking at the reasons why we are still here despite the absence of modern hi-tech medicine being available to our forest dwelling ancestors over thousands of years of their existence on the planet. Evolution of man does not simply follow the naïve Darwinian laws. Environment, in addition, has a lot to do with our evolution. That is seen in many other species as well. One example would suffice. There is a type of butterfly that demonstrates an interesting response upon fleeing from a killer reptile, when pregnant. Upon its escape, it tries to so mutate the offspring's genes that it enables the foetus to develop much larger wing span, making it possible to get away from danger more effectively. The mother butterfly simultaneously mutates the genes of its offspring in the womb to be able to smell the enemy scent from a longer distance, by enhancing the child's olfactory mechanism!

Similar evolutionary changes, based on our environment, kept us going for so long without the assistance of any hi-tech stuff. Let us call this **the intelligence of the body**. Time was when man lived in the forests, and the causes of death were primarily senility or predation. To keep man going despite injury in the likely event of an attack by larger animals, genetic mutation helped to develop the sympathetic system. This could keep one going in an emergency, say bleeding, by redistributing the circulation to supply blood to the vital organs in preference to the non-vital parts and also to help the blood to clot and the bleeding vessels to constrict, arresting blood loss. This friend of man could become his own enemy if used on a long-term basis, as happens in clinical heart failure!

The renin-angiotensin-aldosterone system was another boon to the hunter-gatherer man in the forest, who did not eat extra salt in his food. This prevented his blood pressure from falling to shock levels after injury and bleeding. In the last ten thousand years, the same system has become our curse, with lots of salt added to our diet, resulting in a novel disease, high blood pressure! In Nature, extremes are detrimental. Whereas low sugar-high sugar, low blood pressure-high blood pressure, and low cholesterol-high cholesterol are all bad, constant fluctuations of all these parameters are a must. Stationary levels obtain only after death! The story of man's immune system being able to cope with adversity is also based on the experience of any hostile environment through genetic mutation. History of man in the New World is a good example. When Europeans landed on the American continents the virgin population of that landmass did not have any immunity against the diseases the Europeans were heir to, like small pox. More Natives died due to such scourges than to the European guns.

The Medical world is learning the hard way the need to respect this capacity of the body and not to interfere too much too soon with modern gadgets and powerful drugs, hurting the native wisdom of the body and its in-built protective mechanisms. Some examples would reveal the secret. Our present mindset of "a pill for every ill" and "quick fixes" has to give place to our understanding that there is a self-regulatory compensatory phase inside the human body for every single alteration or accident!

Studies of sex workers in Nigeria and San Francisco have shown that there are many of them in the trade, on a regular basis, housed in the designated areas having "good business", who keep very good health, despite having more than 50% of their clientele with either full blown AIDS or, at least, the presence of the virus in the blood or semen! But the sophisticated classes of sex workers who operate from five-star outfits do not enjoy this immune protection! The same calamity befalls the hapless victim of accidental exposure to AIDS virus! Oxford University has embarked on studies of the Nigerian prostitutes and the healthy ones from San Francisco to see if some sort of vaccine could be produced from the knowledge gained from such sex workers.

Children of migrant workers in Dakshina Kannada district of Indian Karnataka state on the west coast, originally from Northern Karnataka, whose parents do not have lucrative jobs to give them good food, mostly live on makeshift dwellings on the road side literally eating from the dirt, and resist most of the communicable diseases much better than their cousins in clean and rich households! Extra clean surrounding might endanger children's health by exposing them to new risks from ordinarily innocuous germs. Epidemics of viral appendicitis in British primary schools are one such example.

Caucasians exposed to falciparum malaria are likely to die most of the time, if not properly protected by drugs for prevention, as they have not been exposed to this germ earlier. This is due to the lack of racial immunity. Similarly, when Europeans first come to third world countries they usually are not able to tolerate the drinking water that we all take without any harm.

Hostile environments make us acquire the capacity to genetically produce immunity against many adverse situations. The same mechanism could work against us under special circumstances. East Africans living in East Africa have very little, if any, autoimmune diseases. East Africans form the bulk of American blacks. In America they live in a much cleaner environment without exposure to killer germs like malaria, filaria and others found in Africa. The one hundred-fifty odd genes situated in the long arm of the ninth chromosome, exclusively looking after antibody production against invading germs, at times, feel jobless in their new clean surroundings! They could unwittingly manufacture antibodies against body's own cells, resulting in a very high percentage of killer autoimmune diseases in American blacks of East African origin! Strange are the ways of Nature!

Another glaring example appears in a study of the death rate variations in grievously injured soldiers in the Vietnam War vis-à-vis the Falklands War. Whereas helicopter evacuations and immediate blood transfusions and warming were very common during the Vietnam War, during the wintry war in the Falklands those facilities were absent and the wounded soldiers were sometimes left to fend for themselves for long stretches of time in the cold! Curiously, the per capita death in the two groups showed that a much larger number of them survived the wounds in Falklands compared to Vietnam! One would not easily believe this, but this is the bitter truth.

While the body's compensatory mechanisms, discussed above, helped wounded bleeding soldiers on the South American Island front, effectively, the cold weather helped lower the basal metabolic rate thereby lessening the demand for oxygen to the tissues. In Vietnam, the early human intervention with blood transfusion enhanced bleeding by displacing the clot and reducing vasoconstriction, the warmed up body increased the oxygen demand! This kind of mistake occurs many times in some other disease states in the intensive care settings.

Physiological heart failure is another good example. With its onset, the sympathetic system remodels the heart and redistributes circulation, but chronic stimulation makes the same system destroy the heart muscle and enhance failure. If we use blocking drugs at the beginning to knock off the sympathetic system patients could die, but later use of the same drugs, when the body's own protective mechanisms are exhausted, as in clinical heart failure, could save a lot of lives! One could go on and on. Every single intervention by man at the wrong time ends up killing more people than saving them.

It is high time that many of the hi-tech early interventions are properly and meticulously audited in the field before being sold in the market. One would be shocked to know that this does not happen most of the time because of the hype and greed. Newer interventions are touted as the new *avatar* of life-saving-Gods in technological form and are let loose on gullible and demanding patients. It is better to remember the dictum that **while it is the bounden duty of the medical profession to do its best for the suffering humanity, even when knowledge in that field is inadequate, it is a crime to intervene in the healthy segment of the population with newer technology or untried drugs, with the fond hope and assurance of averting long term danger when the latter interventions are not properly audited in that setting.**

Times change and knowledge is bound to change, but *wisdom* lingers on. The prayer of a wise physician of yore, Sir Robert Hutchinson, reveals it all:

God give me deliverance from:
- *not letting the well alone,*
- *treating suffering humans as cases, and*
- *making my treatment worse than his suffering!*

Further Reading

- Hegde BM. *Ancient Wisdom in Health and Science.* 2003, Delhi College of Physicians and Surgeons, New Delhi, India.
- Hegde BM. *You Can Be Healthy.* 2003, MacMillans, India.
- Shervin B Nuland. *Wisdom of the Human Body.*

CHAPTER 4

Societal Health Promotion

Blessed is he who expects nothing; for he will never be disappointed.

—*Jonathan Swift*

I am sure there is no dispute that our society is very sick these days. In fact, in some parts of our great country, the entire society seems to be in the intensive care unit, just about breathing with the help of oxygen and artificial respirators. If the latter are withdrawn, society might even collapse! Even if one comes out of the intensive care unit, at the end of the day, one will still be not completely normal again. It is like mending a broken glass with strong glue. It is broken glass anyway, even after mending. This applies to human life as well. To keep man healthy is our best bet and is very inexpensive too. This applies to societies as well. However good the mending could be, scars of the damage are always there to remind us of the mistakes that we have made in not keeping society intact in the first place. Ever since man started living in groups, on the fertile banks of major rivers in all the continents nearly ten thousand years ago, there have been misunderstandings, wars, misery and pestilence in the world. But to the best of my information there never was a time like ours. The present era could be best described in the paraphrased words of Charles Dickens: The twenty-first century is the best of times if one considers the so-called scientific developments and the worst of times, when one critically looks at human development. Modern civilization, so-called by the western thinkers, is, if anything, bringing man closer to his animal instincts and perhaps even worse. No animal would want to kill another of its species unless forced to do so under special circumstances of hunger. Today, man eats man even when he is fully fed!

Aetiology of the Sickness

What ails human societies all over the world today? **Monetary economy brought all this misery in its wake.** Study of the aboriginal races off the coast of Saskatchewan in Canada, the inhabitants of Innuland, the Innus, shown by their epigraphic history for more than five hundred odd years, gives the clue to the above conclusions. Innus were a strong race of hunter-gatherers and up until 1732 AD they had a sustenance economy where every one of the members was looked after well. This egalitarian set-up got upset when, for the first time in 1732, a Church came to Innuland with the love of God. Dependence started and the next in line was the Williams Company dealing in hides, which taught the Innu to barter his hide for fancy articles like soap, biscuits, etc. To cut a long story short, today every Innu is a Canadian citizen with all the rights and conveniences of other European Canadians, based on their monetary (later plastic card) economy. Innus in their earlier *avatar* did not suffer from any major illnesses and lived far beyond one hundred years. Today, every Innu is heir to all the illnesses, major and minor, that a European Canadian gets—and that too precociously. The only thing that has changed for the Innu is the ravages of a monetary economy in place of the egalitarian sustenance economy. There are other studies done in the US, the Roseto study, for instance, and another done in Chile by Cruz Coke and colleagues, all of which show similar trends. Money, therefore, is the be-all and end-all of human misery. Today, money, with its power, has become our God and making money our religion. To that end in view we have discovered many new methods of hating one another in the name of nationality, region, religion, caste, colour, language, and what have you.

Management of Sickness

As is the practice in modern medicine, and likewise in social matters, we look for quick fix solutions to all our problems. Problems invariably have deep-rooted causes, which never get corrected with these quick fixes. However, the immediate solutions look good on the surface and delude us temporarily. The malady recurs with greater intensity sooner than later. This has been happening each time something serious happens in society. We still do not ponder to think of long lasting solutions to prevent sickness. In medicine also, prevention does not work well when the disease has set in and the process goes on simmering under the cloak of temporary relief, called *palliation* in Latin. Quick fix curative and/or dramatic palliative solutions have not been successful in medicine and will not be successful in any other field.

What Doctors Don't Get to Study in Medical School   13

Be that as it may, let us think of keeping society tranquil and promoting its health. This could only be done through proper education of the future generation. Health of a nation, as the health of an individual, could only be preserved through promotion of a disease-resisting immune system. Proper education of the future generation, giving them the right attitude to life of co-operation and camaraderie alone could keep all of us happy. This new education should start right from day one in school, if not at home, as the child is growing up. In addition to the external, objective, intellect-based knowledge that the present educational system imparts, we have to include internal, intuition-based, subjective knowledge of the self to the child and make him/her realize early on in life that he/she is here to live for others. Truth, ethics, and social responsibilities are to be added on as we go along.

This is fine for another generation, but what will happen to the present generation, most of whom are converts to the hatred ethos that is trying to take the world for a ride in the name of making money? There should be a positive solution for that segment of society as well, lest we should all perish before the new generation takes charge of affairs, armed with the new methods of education.

Let us take our lessons from the other wings of society where similar situations obtain. Let us take the curative medical care system as an example. Time was when a doctor was considered only next to God and the patient had immense faith in the system. That placebo effect was the one that kept us alive on this planet. In fact, analysis shows that in the past such horrible things like animal urine, skin scrapings, metallic ashes, and all kinds of herbs were used in medicine all over the world. Today we claim to have the most scientific remedies! However, audits have consistently showed that the per capita death rate did not appreciably change in the last hundred odd years even though we claim to have methodical remedies and surgical procedures. Rather, they have shown that marginally, we are worse off now.

This is not surprising. Healing of any damage has to be ultimately done by the body's immune system and the best stimulation for that comes from the mind of the sick individual. The latter depends on the patient's confidence in the treating doctor. Technology has taken medicine to the market place, making the doctor a seller of technology and the patient a buyer—a classical monetary economic ethos. With the onset of the consumer movement in medicine, the time honoured doctor-patient relationship has all but vanished, resulting in all types of misery. In many areas, doctors have, in fact, become a menace to society! Recently, doctors went on strike in Israel for three months and the death rate and morbidity statistics went down dramatically, making society much healthier! All these parameters came back to the old levels once doctors came back to work. It is rumored that the morticians are the ones that brokered a peace between the striking doctors and the government as they had very bad business during the strike period.

Let us take a look at the legal field. More the laws in any country, less the justice. Justice delayed, which is the situation now in many countries, is literally justice denied. Civil litigation sometimes takes more than one generation to fructify. Criminal litigation depends on so many extraneous factors that rarely does one get justice. Some cynic recently wrote that if one wants justice one must never go to the courts. This must have been so even in times past. King Ferdinand of France, while sending his people to colonize the newly found Indies in the New World, had one strict rule that no one who has studied jurisprudence should be included in the group, so that the people there at least could live in peace. This may be one of the reasons why our parliament does not function effectively, as most of the honourable members in it are trained in law!

Punishment of crime is another avenue that society uses to treat its maladies. I do not feel that this system has achieved its avowed objectives. A criminal punished becomes a hardened criminal when he comes out of jail. Reformation of the guilty is a more difficult job. In this area, the latest menace seems to be the intolerance that we call terrorism. Each kind of terrorism emanates from some kind of intolerance of another's point of view. It may be in the field of religion, politics or economics but intolerance is where it begins. The Criminal System is not the final answer. It is like bypass surgery for coronary artery disease, palliating the smoking fire within that eventually destroys the whole system. Even the might of the great American nation could not contain Bin Laden's onslaught. A lot of innocent lives get lost in the bargain, just as billions of healthy body cells get destroyed when we burn cancers in the human body with radiation and powerful chemicals!

What is the Remedy?

Having defined the problem let us now think of the solution. The only solution could come from the people themselves. As shown above, any government, police system, army, or judiciary cannot impose the solution. The media and political outfits only aggravate the disease, although the media is supposed to apply a soothing touch. Most of the time, they are so partisan that they incite more trouble as they try to fish in troubled waters to gain some mileage in their struggle for one-upmanship or money.

How does society empower the common man to solve this problem? It can be done by inculcating in him the power of understanding others, using the regular cooperative dialogues between different sections of the society, be it with reference to different religious practices, or settling other disputes without involving any external agency, such as the government, politicians, the media, the judiciary or even the officialdom. Every single village must have a creative dialogue society—call it the Socrates club, if you will—where people meet in the evenings and thrash out their differences (there were many Indian versions of this method but I have refrained from quoting from them lest I should be labeled unprogressive in my thinking). The following Ten Commandments, based on–Socrates clubs elsewhere, should guide them:

- Honour others, and listen to them deeply with all your heart and mind.
- Focus on the agenda while seeking the common ground for consensus, but avoid group-think by acknowledging the diversity of views.
- Refrain from irrelevant and intemperate interventions.
- Acknowledge others' contributions to the discussion before relating your own remarks to theirs.
- Remember that silence also speaks; speak only when you have a contribution to make.
- Identify the critical points of difference for further deliberations.
- Never distort other views to further your own.
- Formulate the agreements on any agenda item before moving to the next.
- Draw out the implications of an agreement for group policy and action.
- Thank everyone for his or her contributions.

Let these Ten Commandments guide our villagers and train them to help themselves. Outside interference of any sort should be prohibited. Let them sort out their differences themselves, as was done by that great philosopher Socrates even in a hostile society. Compassionate dialogue is the only way and the most legitimate weapon for realizing a peaceful society. If this is done on an all-India basis, governments become irrelevant in the common man's life. This will lessen the importance of elections the way we have them now, bringing down the money power of politicians. With that deprivation they will fall to their knees before the people to get their votes. Even voting in any election should be based on this kind of a dialogue for the common good.

The mega projects and the open markets have only impoverished the masses further. We could, through the dialogue method, go back to microeconomic developments of small holding farmers who work together to make agriculture profitable. It is only by developing villages that our country will come out of the bottomless pit into which it has sunk, thanks to the monkey tricks of our politicians and their goons. Non-governmental agencies should come forward to help the poor and the less fortunate. The future belongs to these NGOs. Governments in many countries will have to become irrelevant to the common man's life very soon. The day is not far off when the ordinary man will run his own life without any help from the corrupt powers-that-be. "Cure rarely, comfort mostly but console always" has been the motto of so-called curative medicine. Promotive health is the future of health care delivery. Promotive societal health might save this world from total annihilation.

God! What sort of heart are you going to give us?

—*Anon*

Further Reading

- Hegde BM. *You Can Be Healthy.* MacMillans India, 2004, Delhi.
- Hegde BM. *How to Maintain Good Health?* UBSPD publications, New Delhi. 1993

CHAPTER 5

Health Care–Reaching the Unreached

The difference between the right word and the almost right word in a place is like the difference between lightning and the lightning bug.

—Mark Twain

Health care is a word mostly misunderstood and used in place of palliative medical care. The two are poles apart. It is very important, both for the lay man and the administrators, to make a clear distinction between the two, lest there should be mal-administration of health strategies in society.

Health is a state of holistic wellbeing of man, enabling him to be enthusiastic to be creative in society for his own good as well as for the good of others, the latter more important than the former in the social context. On the contrary, palliative medical care is trying to fix the broken pieces of a healthy man into a whole again. There is further confusion here in that it is sometimes called curative medical care, in place of palliative care. Cure, we rarely, if ever!

If one follows the holistic classification of diseases suggested by me, it would be more practical:

- Emergency medicine (10% of the sick population)
- Minor illness syndromes (around 30%)
- Doctor-thinks-you-have-a-disease (10%)
- Patient-thinks-he-has-a-disease (10%)
- Chronic illness syndromes (remaining 25–30%)
- Drug or doctor induced (iatrogenic) diseases (10–15%)

18 What Doctors Don't Get to Study in Medical School

In this scenario only the first ten per cent of the sick population does need modern hi-tech medical and surgical care. Rest of them could make do with conventional traditional systems of medicine coupled with **changes in the life style.** Modern medicine becomes prohibitively expensive when used for all the one hundred percent of the sick population; it could strain the budget of even the richest nation. America is feeling the pinch. More than sixty percent of the upper middle class Americans can not afford good health cover as the insurance premia are sky high, thanks to the charges of the star-performers. The rest who can afford to pay through their nose can get insurance.

The National Health Service of the UK is broke and the story repeats everywhere. If one were to follow the dictum mentioned above one could give equitable medical care for the really needy. While the American hospitals have been reducing their beds, the new idea of HMOs to replace hospital expenses has not succeeded either.

Action Plan for India for the Next Century

It is true that the population growth in our country is still not arrested while in many western countries it is either decreasing or is, at least, not increasing. They envisage a large chunk of their population in the next millennium to be in the above sixty category (70% of the population). Naturally, they could expect to see degenerative diseases go up exponentially in the west. That would be their real problem. Our scenario would be totally different.

More than sixty per cent of our population in the next millennium would be in the second decade. We would have totally different type of problems of adolescence, viz, AIDS, drug addictions, infective diseases, nutritional disorders, violence, tobacco and alcohol related diseases, and road accident deaths in place of their load of degenerative diseases.

Modern medical wisdom comes in handy here for us to avoid any future threat of degenerative diseases. Most, if not all, degenerative diseases get born in the mother's womb in the first trimester of her pregnancy. It is there that the foetus forms its heart, blood vessels and pancreas, to name a few. These structures, if not formed well, could encourage the onset of heart diseases, high blood pressure, diabetes and other vascular accidents in adult life! It is known now that mother's nutrition in the first trimester of pregnancy is of vital importance to avoid this menace.

What Doctors Don't Get to Study in Medical School

The next period in life when these diseases get their encouragement is childhood and adolescence when bad food habits, alcohol and tobacco could further ensure the progress of degenerative diseases in later life.

Action Plan

1) The comprehensive village development plan should include water supply, toilets, education about common foods available in the village, and also some methods to uplift the economic condition of the villagers. Smokeless choolas should be supplied to all houses.

2) Pregnant mothers should get special attention regarding their diet, more so in the first trimester. Proper nutritional advice should avoid undernourishment during that crucial period in the life of the foetus.

3) Compulsory breastfeeding education to be given to all mothers. In case the breast milk is inadequate, other human milk, if available, is good enough but not cow's milk! Instead, the baby could be given fruit juices and cereals in an easily digestible form. This could avoid many other diseases in later life, like the autoimmune diseases.

4) Effective education, to keep tobacco and alcohol at bay, aimed at the adolescents, using different methods suitable to different set-ups, should be started.

5) Our primary education should change in such a way that it inculcates the essence of Indian education of the yore—humility. Humility begets better life habits. Anger, pride, jealousy, hatred, and ego get suppressed to give place to love, compassion, and camaraderie. The former are now known to be important risk factors for major degenerative diseases.

6) Proper health education of children in school about the dangers of alcohol, tobacco, and also sexually transmitted diseases will go a long way in reducing the future problems of drug addiction and AIDS, which are going to be our big problems in the next millennium.

7) Better roads and stricter licensing procedures should decrease road accident deaths. Coupled with a war on alcohol this should yield better results. The only truly avoidable deaths are accidental deaths. Punishment for careless driving should be more stringent to persuade rich kids from rash driving in larger cities.

8) Family planning should be pursued on a war footing. In the villages, where the bulk of India lives, men are at fault. The best way to educate the men in the village is to catch the village barber. The latter is an incessant talker and also has a lot of influence on all the men in the village. If we could properly educate the barbers and then give them an incentive, that could work wonders in addition to the conventional methods followed.

9) Screening whole populations for high blood pressure, heart disease and diabetes to get them under the net of doctors, drug companies, and instrument manufacturers to fix the defect would look good on paper. It can work in the laboratory, but it does not work in the population, and it is definitely not cost effective.

10) In addition, screening apparently healthy populations could even be counterproductive. "It could seriously damage the health of the population," says Richard Smith, former editor of the British Medical Journal. Past experience has shown that screening increases sick absenteeism in society making more people sick! It also increases false positives.

11) Screening a population of one billion is not feasible. Screening only the urban elite is also not going to help. This would certainly net more people into the system for treatment and also get more hapless victims for intervention in the present top heavy hi-tech medical field, but would not change the scenario as far as the imaginary threat of the degenerative disease epidemics, as predicted. Predicting the future is impossible. "We have been predicting the unpredictable," said Prof. William Firth, a physicist. Reliable studies even in the West have shown that the so-called epidemic rise of certain degenerative diseases and their subsequent fall has been spurious and flawed heavily.

12) Lifestyle modifications have been palpably more effective in containing these diseases even in the West. While the effect of lifestyle modifications has been 59.4% effective in reducing the incidence of coronary artery disease, interventional methods have only been effective to the tune of 3.4%. The story is not different in the field of drug therapy, either. The famous MRC study of mild to moderate hypertension treatment, which has 85,000 patient years of experience, clearly showed that *to save one life from stroke we have to treat 850 apparently healthy people in society with antihypertensive drugs unnecessarily.*

13) Coupled with the prohibitive cost of population screenings and their attendant dangers to human health it makes lot of sense for third world countries to concentrate all their efforts in modifying the lifestyle of their populace to contain these dreaded diseases even if they were expected in the next millennium.

14) Here, the role of *tobacco and alcohol has to be stressed. We have to fight the powers-that-be that try and push these two evils on society, with all our might.*

15) Another area is the field of diet for our adolescents. Indian vegetarian diet has a lot to recommend it to them in place of the modern junk non-vegetarian food, which seems to be invading the world of the young in a big way. Nutrition based education should start in the elementary schools.

16) Need to have physical exercise is the next area to be stressed. This could be done in many ways aimed at the younger generation.

17) The need to keep the human mind filled with universal love to avoid hostility and depression—the two most important risk factors for heart and vessel diseases in addition to cancer—has to be stressed right from day one in school.

18) Economic empowerment of our masses is of vital importance to avoid future epidemics of vascular degenerative diseases.

The need of the hour is the courage to implement these right away and keep the pressures on population screening and mass drugging only to the symptomatic in society, thus bringing down the cost of curative medicine to affordable limits.

Would someone listen please?

> **I'm sick of gruel, and the dietetics,**
> **I'm sick of pills, and sicker emetics,**
> **I'm sick of pulses, tardiness or quickness,**
> **I'm sick of blood, its thinness and thickness-**
> **In short, within a word, I'm sick of sickness!**

—Thomas Hood, *'Fragment',* c. 1844.

Further Reading

- David Barker. *Mothers, Babies, and Chronic Diseases.* 1997. BMA publications, London.
- Stehbens WE. An appraisal of the epidemic rise of coronary heart disease and its decline. *The Lancet* 1987;182: 399–405.
- Brody, Jane and Denise Grady, *The New York Times Guide to Alternative Health.* New York: New York Times Co., 2001. 203–244.
- Stehabens WJ. An appraisal of the epidemic rise of coronary artery disease and its decline. *Lancet* 1987;I: 606–611.
- Stewart-Brown S, Farmer A. Screening could seriously damage your health. *BMJ* 1997; 314: 533–535.

CHAPTER 6

Power of Prayer

I was thrilled to witness a rare phenomenon happening in the holy city of Varanasi on the Mahashivaratri night. Burkha-clad Muslim women were singing bhajans with their brothers and sisters owing allegiance to Lord Shiva. I had tears of joy welling up in my eyes. I still could recall my childhood in our village where people of all religions, Christians and Muslims included, joined us in celebrating, not only the religious festivals but, also, the village rituals like the buffalo race, Bhoota kola, etc., common to coastal Karnataka. We, on our part, used to share in their joy and also partake in their wonderful food on Easter, Christmas, Bakrid and Moharam days. I grew up not knowing that we have any difference whatsoever. The environment now makes me feel nauseated to say the least, but those Mahashivaratri night TV clippings were a great relief. How I wish all of us could take it forward from there.

Coincidentally, the occasion was the right one. Though the rituals were meant to pray to the all-powerful Shiva that night, the connotation was to try and open one's third eye, representing the third eye of Lord Shiva. The third eye is the symbolic representation of one's ability to see the reality. The two eyes, which most of us have, with or without artificial corrections using lenses, could only show us the world of delusion. Very rarely a few of us have evolved to have our third eye function to have an insight into another's sorrow to be able to empathize with him/her. One is supposed to fast that night, sit-up and pray to Lord Shiva to grant us the power of the symbolic third eye (the insight) to be able to see the reality in this world. "Purusha Shreshta Ishwaraha." One could elevate oneself to that level by spiritual efforts.

The reality is that mankind is but one large family and God is only the all pervading universal compassion that gives succor to every living thing on this planet. We might create our own individual Gods and there is no harm in that. We always create God in our own image. But none of our Gods would want us to be at each other's throats using HIS name. God and conventional religions should strive to bring man and man together and never try to divide man from man. All right thinking people would support this contention that religion is meant to be social shock absorber.

Religion, initially created to bring tranquility and contentment to the human mind, has unfortunately, over the years, become a powerful tool to have control over the gullible people. When one tries to understand one's religion thoroughly, he/she would automatically love another human being outside his own narrow religious beliefs. With this in view, one should strive to use ritualistic religion to bring people together. Every one in this world, has an obligation to see that this world becomes a better place to live in— more tranquil, more passionate, more productive and less destructive in the end. Intolerance of any kind is the beginning of terrorism and crime. Tolerance needs more giving than getting.

At a more mundane level, this philosophy boils down to using all our religious festivals to bring about inter-religious harmony. Whereas there were bhajans in the temples on the Mahashivaratri day joined in by the Muslim women, there could be prayers in Churches during Christmas and large gathering of people in the Mosques on Muslim festival days. On each of those occasions there must be more people from the other religions in these group prayers. Scientific studies have shown that intercessory prayers have a very powerful positive effect on the life and health of human beings. If each one of us in the community prays for the welfare of the people of other religious beliefs, we would certainly have a society, which would be more creative and caring but less destructive.

Mankind has been happy in the sustenance economies of the distant past where there was no dependence of any kind coupled with egalitarian sharing and caring for others. Fear of God, greed for money, and running after the mirage of power has slowly turned man into a cruel animal. Love of God would undo this cycle for certain. Today, man does not even bat an eyelid to destroy another of his species in the name of religion, caste, creed and what have you.

We must try to garner the strengths of good people in society to do most good to most people most of the time. In every village, town and city we could organise groups of motivated citizens from all religions to implement the idea that they should live together and let live. One of the cementing factors could be this type of interfaith prayer meetings. On the days of the important festivals in temples, people from other religions could be invited to sing bhajans and take part in the ceremonies. Similarly during Christmas, Easter time other religious segments should be there in the churches for prayers and the mass. Islamic festivities should be co-sponsored by other religious adherents and all should visit Mosques with our Muslim brothers in their neighbourhood.

Recently, when I was in Mumbai, I enjoyed the bhajans of a group of people who came from very far off coastal Karnataka. They sang and danced so well that it was a moving spectacle to watch. How I wish they had invited people of all faiths to share in their joys that day. Majority of people in this world are good but silent. It is a vocal minority, which creates problems for others. By and large, people are nice to one another if left to themselves. When politicians and others manipulate them with ulterior motives society gets disturbed. It is always better to debate on contentious issues like this rather than to accept or reject an idea without any debate. Let these thoughts provoke an active debate all over. I am sure the powers-that-be swould sit up and take note of the happenings.

Intellectual intolerance is the worst kind of terrorism. Poverty and illiteracy will breed terrorists, in addition. Well-meaning citizens should take up the cause of the less fortunate in society to try and assist them to come out of the bottomless pit of poverty. It cannot be done in bits and pieces. This must be a large movement on a large nationwide scale. Misguided youth, with lots of energy and wrong directions from the vested interests, initially try to be destructive for the heck of it. Eventually, it becomes a part of their lifestyle and they get inured to all the dangerous fall-outs. At that stage, punishment need not (usually does not) have long-term good effects on society. Prevention is always better.

Poverty has one other flip side to it. The poor pay for their poverty with their lives. Poverty is also the mother of all human illnesses. How do we expect these people to come to the mainstream of society, unless those of us who are above the poverty line come out with a helping hand? In this process we are not doing any favour to the poor people. We are only doing our duty to society. We are helping Gods of all religions to help those in distress. As a bonus we are improving our health. Molecular biology tells us that when one tries to help others the immune system gets a shot in the arm to get stronger.

The present set-up cannot be allowed to go on like this and eventually lead to anarchy. Please think about it with all seriousness. Man has existed here for nearly nine hundred thousand years in fifty thousand generations. The present cruel world might have been there for a maximum of one hundred years. If not corrected soon enough, greedy man, with his proclivity for personal comfort would rob the world and the less fortunate people of the entire God given resources. Let us wake up to stop this rot before it takes deeper roots. You would wonder now as to the role of doctor in all these. Doctors are trained to keep the health of society and social tranquility is a pre-requisite to good health of the masses. We, doctors, therefore should be in the forefront of this movement for tranquility. This is not taught to you in the medical school!

FURTHER READING

- Hegde BM. The unrest cure. *J Assoc Physi India.* 1997; 47: 730–731.
- Whiteman MC, Fowkes FGR, Deary IJ. Hostility and the Heart. *BMJ* 1997;315:379–81.
- Rose G (2001) Sick individuals and sick populations. *Int J Epidemiol* 30: 427–432.
- Department of Health (2004 November) *Choosing health: Making healthier choices easier.* CM 6374 London: The Stationary Office. 207 p.

CHAPTER 7

The Art of Medicine

> I keep six honest serving me,
> They have taught me all I know.
> Their names are, who, why, where,
> What, when and how.
>
> —*Rudyard Kipling*

I do not remember why I wanted to be a doctor in the first place, but doctor I did become like any one of you and was as proud and arrogant as any one could be until, once upon a time nearly thirty years ago, I was called to see a young man of thirty brought dead to our coronary care unit, in the wee hours of the morning. The most profound question that the young widow asked me, clutching my ankles, shook me from my deep slumber: "Why did my husband die, doctor?" For the first time in my life my intellectual impotence came to light. I could have given her a big lecture on how her husband died, but not why!

Charles Sherrrington, a great physiologist, was appointed professor of physiology at the University of Liverpool, at the age of 42, in the year 1899. While delivering his acceptance speech he said, "Positive sciences cannot answer the question "Why". They can, at best, answer "How" or "How much", but never why! A physiologist could say how does the heart contract but would never be able to say why does the heart contract."

That took me to philosophy, religion, theology, teleology, and what have you! The one book that gave some comforting thoughts was the Penguin classic written in 1927 by a great American novelist, Thornton Wilder: *The Bridge on San Luis Rey*. The book has an explanation to comfort the relatives of the dead. It talks about the world of the living and the world of the dead. The two are connected by an unbreakable bridge of human lives. So one continues to consider the dead as if they are still here. This is quite comforting. Life and death are not in our hands. Let us not take the public for a ride by claiming that we could save people from the jaws of death. This kind of self aggrandizement has now landed us in the market place with consumerism getting into this arena of doctor-patient trust, the one that kept us going from the time of God Dhanvanthari. The mutual trust is the apex of medical care. The crucial part of medicine is the coming together of two human beings, the one who is ill or imagines he/she is ill and the one in whom the former has confidence. This is necessary for the human immune system to get stimulated **to heal the malady.**

The Art of Medicine

Listening to the patient is the most difficult part of a doctor's life. Learn to listen and you will succeed as a good doctor. Listening is the first and foremost part of the whole gamut of doctor-patient relationship. Healing is an art. The healer must master his technique just as a painter does. A good doctor should master the art of healing, never becoming so lost in the western obsession with objectivity and its emphasis on reproducibility of experimentation. Empirical wisdom could help a good doctor to the same extent, if not more, than the so-called evidence-based medicine. There are several problems with the evidence of the evidence-based medicine. Many times the modern medicine becomes evidence burdened instead of evidence based. The art of healing is not being taught in medical schools in most countries. The pity is that even in the Indian Ayurvedic system, the mother of all systems of healing, taught in Indian schools of Ayurveda, we seem to have forgotten this important part of education of a doctor. We teach medical students to listen, palpate, auscultate, and scan, but forget to tech them the most important ingredient of human affairs: to *feel* pain, disability, and suffering of another human being; in short, to have an insight into another's sorrow. Unless a doctor learns to feel other's pain, he/she would never understand what it is to suffer from pain and how important it is for him/her to ease the other person's pain! Learning to feel other's pain is the main part of a doctor's education. Henry David Thoreau wrote, "to affect the quality of the day - that is the highest of arts." Medicine has the capacity to affect the quality of the day for the hapless patient. Let us remember it for the rest of our lives. To be a good doctor is the greatest opportunity in life as it is the only way one gets exposed to human emotions in their pristine glory and virginity.

Qualities of Head and Heart

One of the essential qualities of the clinician is interest in humanity, for the secret of the care of the patient is in caring for the patient.
—*Francis Weld Peabody, 1881–1927.*

Doctors need two special qualities of the head and heart that make them *placebo* doctors and therefore good healers:

1) **Imperturbability:** Under no circumstances of peace or war you should get perturbed while dealing with patients. Your body language, even a frown, could kill an anxious patient.

2) **Aequanimitas:** Keep your mental cool under all trying situations, come what may. It needs a cool mind to rationally think in an emergency situation.

A good doctor could be compared *"to the promontory on the sea, against which, though the waves beat continually, yet it both stands, and about it are those swelling waves stilled and quieted",* as enunciated by Marcus Aurelius.

Medicine as a Business

Medicine, riding piggyback on technology, has gone to the market place in a big way. This has destroyed medical ethics, making most of us hypocrites swearing by the Hippocratic Oath! Even research is no longer the measure of honesty and purity. There are enough and more studies showing that the so-called evidence-based medicine is really evidence burdened, in favour of drug companies and technology manufacturers. Doctors are being bought over by both drug companies and instrument manufacturers to sell their wares.

"*Is Academic Medicine for Sale?"* is an editorial in a recent issue of the *New England Journal of Medicine* (2000; 342:1516) and *Medical Education in the US is run by Drug Company Money* is the caption of an editorial in *The Lancet (2000; 356: 781).* Cardiac procedures are done more to get money than to help the patient is the essence of an editorial in the *NEJM* (1997, page 1523). I have only given you a sample of the rot that has already set in. Writing a book *Science without Sense* (CATO Institute, Washington, 1999) Steven Milloy shows how medical research is faked deliberately many times!

A senior teacher of medicine, Frank Davidoff, who also was the editor of the *Annals of Internal Medicine* for well over thirty years, laments in his book *Who Has Seen A Blood Sugar (1997 ACP publications, Philadelphia)* how we try and treat the blood reports and neglect the suffering human being, the owner of the report: the latter many times suffers more by our interventions. He calls this as *euboxic medicine*. As long as the computer boxes are all correctly ticked, doctors do not worry about patients in defensive medicine.

Remember that all that glitters is not necessarily gold even in science.

I shall recommend that you keep this prayer of a great **clinician**, Sir Robert Hutchinson, on your work table:

God, give us deliverance from:
- Not letting the well alone
- Treating human beings as cases, and
- Making our interventions worse than his disease

How true!

You are still non-converts, I hope. Keep medical science as pure as you possibly could. Try to change the trend if you could; but remember that you would be up against the stone wall in this area.

> **Fear not! Life still**
> **Leaves human effort scope.**
> **But, since life teems with ill,**
> **Nurse no extravagant hope.**
> —Mathew Arnold. *Empedocles on Etna*

Money is not the criterion to judge you as a good doctor. Never try and make money in the sick room. You will get your due and, a fair share at that. Do not be in a hurry to make it big fast: no one has taken money with him while going at the end of life! The gratitude and the smile on the face of a grateful patient are priceless and give you true happiness. One must strive to earn such smiles in abundance.

Some of you will fail in life, but never lose heart. It is in losing that you win. "From our desolation only does the better life begin," advised Sir William Osler. If you can treat triumph and disaster, the two imposters, just the same, you will come on top.

Your Alma Mater

While the West was still dwelling in the forests, we in India had Universities of excellence attracting scholars from all over the then civilized world. Be proud of your Alma Mater. Universities are not judged by their pride, pomp, and circumstances, nor their wealth, number of schools or halls, but by the *men and women*, your teachers, who have trodden in its service the thorny road through toil. Remember them all and also your Alma Mater in times of prosperity. Many foreign Universities depend on the munificence of their alumni. Do not let your University down.

Complementary Systems of Medicine

Modern hi-tech medicine has become so prohibitively expensive that today even 62% of the upper middle class Americans cannot afford health insurance in that country. 57% of Britons would want to opt out of the system, if they could. *While the ten percent of emergency quick-fix measures depend only on modern medicine, one could do well to avoid modern medicine in non-emergency chronic illness scenario, as also in minor illness syndromes that form the bulk of health care delivery problems to make medical care available to all sufferers. Many of our quick-fix methods in emergency care, however, are still to be audited for their efficacy!* (*Chest* 1999; 115:857)

One could practice allopathy, homeopathy, or any other pathy successfully, if only one could combine that with sympathy and empathy in good measure. Health care would be possible for the poor masses if we teach our students the significance of taking the best from all the complementary systems, in a judicious mix, keeping the touchstone of scientific methods at the centre of our choice. In this area, Ayurveda, the mother of all systems of health care, stands out as the most scientific and effective. One must, however, understand that Ayurveda is not synonymous with herbal medicines. It is the science of life and living.

With quantum physics opening the eyes of the modern scientists to the beauties of the human mind (consciousness) in human illnesses, interest in Ayurveda, which has been proclaiming to the world for centuries the prime role of the mind in diseases, has been recognized as the best and the most scientific. Heisenberg's *Uncertainty Principle* and Schrodinger's *Cat Hypothesis* have endeared scientists to the holistic science of Ayurveda.

32 What Doctors Don't Get to Study in Medical School

Ever since medicine was accepted as a science in the European Universities in the twelfth century, medicine relied on linear mathematics. Linear mathematics does not hold good in dynamic systems like the human body. "Doctors have been predicting the unpredictable," says William Firth, a physicist in Glasgow (*BMJ* 1991 26th Dec. issue). We have also been frightening people by picking out numerous risk factors like the magician pulling out pigeons from his hat. If one were to avoid all the so-called risk factors one cannot possibly live on this earth. Most, if not all of them, cannot predict the outcome as time evolves. All that was explicitly explained in the time-honoured wisdom of Ayurveda.

Continuing Medical Education

The Sanskrit etymological root of the word "physician" is "*bheu*" which means *to grow*. It is now time for you to *unlearn* what you had learnt so far for the examinations and *re-learn* the real life medicine to do most good to most people most of the time. *Let not your medical schooling come in the way of your education!* Keep learning as long as you live. Human knowledge changes faster than you think. Most of us would not know what has changed under our very nose, if we do not keep in touch. One must learn from one's mistakes. It is totally wrong to believe that doctors do not and cannot commit mistakes. If that were true, doctors would be doing nothing. Do not get frustrated if you commit any mistake, but do take care that you never ever repeat the same mistake twice! Never sweep your mistakes under the carpet. Grow from your mistakes to be a better doctor; so-called **anubhooti**.

In conclusion, I admit that all cannot achieve greatness but try one must. If we aim at the sky we would certainly reach the first floor.

**Manushaanaam Sahareshu, Kashcid yathaathi Siddaye,
Yataamapi Siddaanaam Kaschin maam vetti tattvathaha.**
—*Bhagawad Gita*

(When thousand people try one might reach excellence, but when thousand such excellent people struggle one would reach me [the top])

> I have striven all my life,
> Not to **HATE** human action,
> Not to **LAUGH** at human action,
> Not to **WEEP** at human action,
> But to **UNDERSTAND** human action.
>
> —*Spinoza*

FURTHER READING

- Milloy Steven. *Science without Sense.* 1997, Cato Institute, Washington DC.
- Richard Smith. *Medical Journals as the extension of Drug Company influence.* PLOSmedicine 2005
- Starfield Barbara. Is the US medicine the best in the world? *JAMA* 2000; 284: 483–485.

CHAPTER 8

The Fine Art of Living

*The ear says more
Than any tongue.*

—WS Graham, *The Hill of Intrusion*

Living is an art, and a fine art at that. "Art is that which makes the man's day," said Henry David Thoreau. I quite agree with him. While we teach all sorts of unwanted facts to our children at school, making life miserable for them during examinations as they try to recall them all, we never make an attempt to train them in the art of living, which is what they have to do for the rest of their lives. It reminds me of the old saying that we teach our students British history and Indian history but never their family history, the latter might be more useful even if taught at home. Consequently, most children learn the art of living by living life experimenting and imitating others, mostly their parents at home and teachers and peers in school. Many of us elders are anything but good examples.

Man's ingress into this world has always been naked and bare; his egress from this world is also out of his control. He does not even know when, how, and where he will exit. The period in-between is what he has control over. If that bit could be made happier, he would have lived well. "Our progress in this world is trouble and care," wrote DH Lawrence. **Trouble is an integral part of living, but care is what makes it worth living.** How do we go about our daily routine caring for others? This act of caring for others is the art of living, nay the fine art of living. Getting more and more does not make one happy, as man always wants more; but giving makes one always happy. The art of giving is the art of living.

What Doctors Don't Get to Study in Medical School

Let us look at some of the best examples of this hypothesis. Bill Gates, the richest American, gave away a whopping sum of one billion dollars, the biggest individual charity in history, but not for nothing. He must have earned the goodwill of the world and thereby happiness for himself! Nelson Rockefeller Sr. was a very successful Texan billionaire, at the young age of fifty-two. He pulverized every other man in the oil business and earned a lot of enemies. His effigies were burnt every day. He could not go out without bodyguards. With all that he was not happy. He fell into a strange distemper. He lost twenty pounds in weight, had lost his appetite completely, and was not getting a wink of sleep at night. He looked ill and old in his middle age. One of those sleepless nights in bed gave him the solution to his problem as all the doctors and technology in America, could not help him. Early the following morning he went to see his lawyer to establish the Rockefeller Foundation. He completely recovered and went on to live into his eighties, healthy and happy. Alfred Nobel earned a fortune selling dynamite, which he had invented. He was the richest European of his time. Following a mysterious fire in his factory, which Alfred survived with the skin of his teeth, he changed completely, giving away his last Swiss Frank for a total of 800 million to create the Nobel Prize Trust; Alfred lived happily ever after!

Jamshedjee Tata, JRD Tata, GD Birla and many other Indian businessmen did the same to get happiness. Most business houses have their charities. The more you give the more you get by way of happiness. Durgadas Mandelia has established a Trust for helping the less fortunate, the Janatha Janardhan Trust. All these and many more have come out of the joy of living for others that these infracaninophiles realized during their lifetimes.

The other thing that makes life miserable is the "I" concept, the super ego. Let us examine this concept scientifically. Every single cell in the human body, of which there are about one hundred thousand billion in all, likes the other cells so much that it is difficult to keep cells away from one another. Even when cells die due to any disease, other cells in the vicinity slip to take their place. This *cell slipping* is a very important aspect of remodeling of organs after illness. In fact, our body cells love the cells in other human and animal bodies so much that all living things would have fused into a large sheet of cells if *Nature* had not invented the mechanism of *immunity*. We would have been one large sheet of body cells in this Universe, called the *syncitium*. If that were the philosophy of the human cell how could we as human beings hate one another or think that we are superior to another person?

Many of us suffer from the unhappiness of feeling that we are very powerful and all others should be subservient to us. This also is unscientific.

Inside every cell in our body there are the battery chargers that run us and make us do every bit of what we do. We walk, talk, laugh, or even lift our little finger because of those batteries. Those batteries—the basal bodies, centrioles and the mitochondria—are not all human organ parts. They belong genetically to an outside germ! During the millions of years of evolution they swam into our original *procaryocyte* long before it became the *eucaryocyte*. Man is rented, hired, or fired as they wish. Where then is the power that people think they possess? It is all a big myth!

Many of us suffer indignities, imaginary losses, and lose our cool because of our imaginary empires. Even the mother earth that we inhabit looks smaller than a speck of dust when viewed through Hubble's telescope with reference to the macrocosm. What of our empires then? All this should make us humbler by the day. Humility is the essence of true education and is lacking in the present system of education. The competitive ethos that we imbibe from our educational system makes us proud and arrogant to think that we are very powerful and could move mountains. The fact still remains that humility gives one peace of mind and happiness.

Quantum physics has made conventional wisdom in sciences look like child's play. It has turned all our concepts about solid states and matter upside down. Nothing in this Universe is solid. Every atom in its core consists of waves of hydrons rotating at phenomenal speeds and held by the enormous force of attraction to the nucleus. That is why we get atomic energy when we bombard an atom. The apparent solidity of the human body or a tabletop is an illusion. Just as a fan, when run very fast, looks like a sheet of metal instead of different leaves, the illusion of solidity comes from the speed of motion of the hydrons around an atomic nucleus. Every aspect of this Universe described is eventually in the eye of the beholder!

When one goes still further, the last bits of every atom are the *lepto-quarks*. They are so subtle that they cannot be perceived easily. They are identical in all of us and they could even exchange from one to another. The ancient Indian concept of *Satsanga* comes from this concept. Good company gets you good lepto-quarks and vice versa. Even the adage *"birds of the same feather flock together"* must have come from years of observational research in society.

Man has very little scientific basis to think that he is all-powerful. United, men are very powerful; divided, they fall very soon. It is in everyone of our own interest to be helping one another. Happiness is in giving and sorrow is in store while getting. One could see the dire need to be charitable in life. All of us cannot be Bill Gates to be giving away money. The greatest charity in life is not giving money, food, or blood. One could do a lot of good to society if one could be charitable to spare another man one's judgement. Judging others and passing our judgement could be the most painful experience for the recipient. All of us could practise this charity. That is, in fact, giving our love to one and all. The real art of living is loving one another!

One other aspect of unhappiness in life is our emotional reaction to life situations. When we get angry and react to our anger it is some chemical in our body that is making us do what we do. Anger, depression, jealousy, pride, contempt for others, our false sense of superiority and every other human emotion is the handiwork of some chemical or the other inside our system. This is akin to a drunken man talking and behaving abnormally under the influence of alcohol. Just as alcohol temporarily converts man into a monkey, these chemicals, *catecholamines* and related compounds, make a monkey of an emotionally upset man. Once this realization dawns on us, we feel ashamed to react to our emotions. When we do not react to our emotions abnormally we have no reason to be unhappy.

What then are the secrets of the fine art of living? Universal love, compassion, sparing another of our judgement, not abnormally reacting to human emotions, and filling our minds with good thoughts for good deeds for others are in essence the ingredients of the potion for happiness.

One has also to remember that if we did all this and kept quiet, our mouths will not be fed from heaven. Man is made to work. Work is worship. Work never kills. Laziness might kill. Work one must, very hard at that, but with total detachment from self-aggrandizement. Results, good or bad, under those circumstances do not bother us. If one loves one's work one does not feel tired. Make your work your play and enjoy working. Most of us do a job for salary, which is tiresome. Very few of us know the art of working, which is done for love of working. Rewards will come automatically. Making a fast buck quickly requires devious means to achieve success, but decent living and enjoying life is possible with sincere authentic work.

Life is a challenge. One must meet the challenge with courage of conviction. The fine art of living is living for others! This is the first lesson a doctor should learn in the medical school.

If neither foes nor loving friends can hurt you,
If all men count with you, but none too much;
If you can fill the unforgiving minute
With sixty seconds' worth of distance run,
Yours is the Earth and everything that's in it,
And - which is more-you'll be a Man, my son!

—Rudyard Kipling (1865–1936)

Further Reading

- Norman Cousins. *Anatomy of an Illness.* 1979. Norton and Company Inc. NewYork.

CHAPTER 9

Doctors' Dilemma

>Oh! let us never, never doubt
>What nobody is sure about!
>
>—*Hilaire Belloc* (1870–1953)

A thinking doctor will have a great dilemma in the midst of all the medical claptrap that is being sold to the gullible public. Most of what we do is not being properly audited: when audited, the bench marks used are questionable. The euboxic medicine, trying to see that all the boxes in the computer generated case records are filled to avoid future litigation, practised in the west today and copied by others would only keep the record sheets straight but might result in dysboxic death, death at unexpected time and place, of the patient! This is one of the reasons why the death and disability rates went down when doctors went on strike in Israel in 2000. This has to change and the earlier it happens the better for humankind.

Our present disease-based medical education should be replaced by patient (human) oriented medical education of yore where the patient was the kingpin in the game of healing. Great brains of the past— Thomas Lewis, Sir William Osler, Lord Platt, Sir George Pickering, Paul Wood, Paul Dudley White, Sam Levine, Thomas Holme Sellers, Lord Brock, Lord Brain, John Hutchinson and many other thinkers of the past—had said this time and again but we, in our present delusion with scopes and scanners thought that we need not pay heed to these people. In fact, if one re-reads that classic by Richard Asher, *Talking Sense,* even today one would wonder that his writings are so contemporary and very topical. They all had robust common sense, which is a scarce commodity in the medical world today.

Lord Platt wrote: "If you listen to your patient long enough he/she would tell you what is wrong with him/her." Today's technologists would think this is madness. However, a recent double blinded, prospective, computerized study in London showed that *listening to the patient and reading the referral letter gave 80% of the accurate final diagnosis and one hundred per cent of the idea of future management strategies in medical out-patient diagnosis.* Would not this cost a lot less?

Value-based medical education, preferably based mainly in the community, would solve some of the problems, like over-investigation and over-treatment that result in many Ulysses syndromes. Rather, teaching in the hi-tech set up should be discouraged to make the doctor-patient relationship the sheet anchor of medical care delivery. Medical students should have lessons in medical humanism, which includes insight into the real health problems and their solutions. Research must be better regulated. Financial interests of the researchers need to be carefully assessed before publishing their data. Time is now ripe for openness in research.

The profession, before being advertised to the gullible public, should evaluate newer heroic surgical feats that bring in fame, money and status to doctors, hospitals and the vendors of equipment. Deportation of the physician under the most draconian law in South Africa, in the much publicized first heart transplant, for refusing to declare the donor brain dead, is a glaring example of what happens behind the scenes in such situations. We need stricter control over these heroic procedures where the real hero is the patient who offers himself for the procedure unaware of its implications and hazards. Interventions could be audited, like drugs, by controlled studies. Many new techniques had resulted in mortality and morbidity in the past: they are too many to enumerate! Most of them have been swept under the carpet.

Medicine revolves round anxiety—patient anxiety of disability and death and doctor anxiety of having done enough of the right thing or not. If something could be done to allay both these, we will have progressed in the right direction. Doctor's dilemma that causes so much of stress related diseases among doctors goes unnoticed to the detriment of patients and the public. This has to be urgently addressed by the profession as also the powers-that-be. This is not a small matter. Hope sanity will prevail and medical education gets suitably modified with special stress on continued rounded professional development of the practitioners.

Before society loses faith in doctors we have to change for the better and make modern medicine accessible to the majority of the suffering humanity. The popularity of complementary systems is not to be taken lightly despite the fact that we shout from house tops day in and day out that complementary systems are not scientific, people in large numbers opt for those systems. They are not fools to do so. Let us introspect before it is too late. *We should remember that a patient could live without we doctors but doctors cannot live without patients.* Before we reach that stage let us act wisely and set our house in order.

> **Man's mind stretched to a new idea never goes back to its original shape.**
> —*Oliver Wendell Holmes*

Further Reading

- Richard Asher. *Talking Sense.* 1952, BMA Publications, London.
- Shervin B Nuland. *Wisdom of the human body.* 1993. Connecticut.
- Hegde BM. *Ancient Wisdom in Science and Health.* 2003. Delhi College of Physicians and Surgeons. Orange Dot Publishers. Delhi.

CHAPTER 10

Joys and Sorrows
(Job Stress Management)

> I have striven all my life, not to weep at human actions,
> Not to laugh at them, not to hate them,
> But to understand them.
> —*Spinoza,* the Spanish Philosopher

Every job in this world comes with its in-built joys, and associated sorrows. It is only that person who could look at both these imposters alike that enjoys all the seasons of life; the cold of winter, the heat of summer, and the warmth of the spring. Those who have not learnt the art of living with joys and sorrows always complain and suffer from distress.

For the conventional physiologist, like the Late Canadian Professor, Hans Selye, stress meant a series of stereotyped responses of the animal endocrine system to the various stressors in life. He had done a lot of work in this field. The common man's meaning of stress is marginally different. Caplan defines stress from the psychiatrist's point of view: **"It is to denote the collective gamut of anxieties and pressures of the job, the impetus to seek promotion and success, the desire to avoid failure at any cost, the increasing demands of the post, and more, have all been bundled into the word `stress,' in general."** Another excellent viewpoint is that given by Lazarus and Folkman who defined stress **"as a particular relationship between the person and the environment that is appraised by the person as taxing or exceeding his or her resources and endangering his or her well being."**

Stress, no longer means the simple word that it is, but always denotes the pathological connotation attached to it. Hans Selye makes this distinction when he talks about 'stress' and 'distress.' Stress, in the normal sense of the word, is an integral part of life itself. There is no life without stress. If one could avoid all stresses in life, he would wither away and die. Stress is the normal stimulus for growth. That said, I must mention that it is the abnormal reaction to stress that makes man suffer in the end. The title of this chapter might amuse some of you, but the fact is that joys and sorrows could both be equally stressful. Marriage and divorce are shown to be equally stressful, in elegant scientific studies. That is why I called them imposters both, following the footsteps of Rudyard Kipling, when he, in his poem "*If*", said:

> **If you can meet with triumph and disaster,**
> **And treat those two imposters just the same**

He goes on to give tips for stress management in life in the following lines, in addition:

> **If you can keep your head when all about you**
> **Are losing theirs and blame it on you,**
> **If you can trust yourself when all men doubt you,**
> ....
> **If you can wait and not be tired of waiting,**
> **Or being lied about, and don't deal in lies,**
> **Or being hated, and don't give way to hating,**
> ....
> **If you can talk with crowds and keep your virtue,**
> **Or walk with Kings-nor lose the common touch,**
> ....
> **Yours is the Earth and everything that's in it,**
> **And- which is more-you'll be a Man, my son!**

This poem, which netted the highest votes in a recent poll to decide the best English poem, tells us all about the joys and sorrows of any job, nay any life situation.

The concept of *swadharma* in the Bhagavad-Gita, in the present context, talks about the situation of job stress and its management. Strictly speaking, *swadharma* is work according to one's nature (wrongly interpreted by some in the past as the work related to one's birth in the Varna system of society). In today's society this may be impossible to achieve. The real meaning of *swadharma* is to work with dedication. If it is found that the work allotted is not to one's liking, one could try and change it into a new one, called *paradharma*. Ultimately, if one agrees to do a particular job, he has to do it with the feeling that he is not doing it just for the remuneration, but doing it as an offering to God with detachment. The latter gives satisfaction and also peace of mind needed to avoid day-to-day stresses.

Indian scriptures give a lot of information on stress management in particular, and administration, in general. Awareness of these could make us grow *vertically,* while the western techniques in management let us grow only *horizontally.* Many of the best management institutes in India, and a few in the West, have taken note of these far reaching methods, which not only try to give the student an idea of how to manage with the head, but to give an inkling into management from the heart. It is only those who have the ability to combine a strong head with a large heart that could be ideal administrators. This could look preposterous for the novice, but is a sublime philosophy of life according to Jesus Christ who said: **"Be ye, therefore, wise like a serpent, but harmless like a dove".**

Martin Luther King Jr. was of the opinion that when militancy could be combined with humility, the world would be a better place to live in. How sublime are these thoughts, culled from various sources, at different times in history of mankind. Man does not change! Shakespeare was of the opinion that: **"Man in a cottage or castle, palace or pad, is governed by the same emotions and passions."** Introspection is one such method advocated by the Indian wisdom of yore, where each sorrow could be analyzed to make the administrator better suited to deal with similar human problem, the next time. This is called **anubhoothi,** in contrast to, **anubhava (experience).** The psychological change that the administrator undergoes, in the bargain, is the essential element in his or her real growth; the latter is vertical, as noted above.

Just as there are no problems without human beings involved, there can never be any sorrow (problem) without a psychological background to it. If there is no problem in administration there is no joy in the job. There is a beautiful motto in a London primary school, which goes thus: **"Happiness is living dangerously."** I did not believe in this until I took up an administrative post in our organization. I have now come to believe that every problem (sorrow) is an opportunity with thorns on it. If you learn to remove the thorns carefully, you can always cash in on the opportunity underneath. That needs a deep study of human psyche, because man is what he thinks he is.

When one goes to the root of the word **psyche** one understands this concept better. The word psyche has Greek roots. The allegoric representation goes back to the soul (psyche, in Greek) being immortal. Psyche (pronounced psychee—all Greek words that end with an e are pronounced with ee) was supposed to be the name of the most beautiful woman on earth, at the time. She earned the wrath and envy of Aphrodite, not only because she was very beautiful, but also because she was the beloved of Aphrodite's most handsome son, Eros. Aphrodite, who put three most difficult obstacles on her way, made life impossible for her. Finally, she had to be rescued by other Gods, to be eventually reunited with her beloved, Eros.

All this looks fine! But our ancient wisdom has it that we do our duty more to satisfy our inner God. One could cheat anyone on this earth, but not his own conscience, the indwelling God. As administrators, our greatest boss should be our own conscience. Nothing is permanent here on earth, except the good that we do to others. When an administrator understands this, his sorrows get converted into his joys. This, I found, was the best stress management technique. What good could one do while on this earth, better than trying to help another human being in distress? Most of our sorrows in office are egocentric. If one could win over his ego, life becomes a perpetual joy. This inner God of ours, our conscience, should be our guide in all our actions, who is omnipresent, but being subtle cannot be perceived easily. We can never escape his keen observations. All sorrows administrators are heir to, like ego, corruption, pride, anger, jealousy, arrogance disappear once one understands this philosophy.

Many institutes have regular **Yoga** sessions for their departmental and institutional heads to make them tranquil. Yoga should not be misunderstood to be synonymous with aasanaas. " **Chitta vritti nirodhah yogaha.**" **Yoga is controlling the mind and making man more tranquil in his dealings with others. Our real boss is there everywhere around us:**

> **Bahir Anthascha Bhootanaam Achram Charaam eva ch,**
> **Sookshmaavath tad avijneyam doorastham cha antikecha tat**
> That which is both inside and outside everything, it is moving, yet stationary. As it is very subtle it cannot be perceived by senses; it looks far, yet is very near.
> —*Bhagavad Gita*

The word stress now has a medical connotation, in addition. This refers to the 'burn-out', a term coined by Freudenberger in 1974, to describe "the demoralization, disillusionment, and exhaustion that results from work in **those stressed by wrong attitudes to work"**. Now that word has been elevated to a diagnostic label in the WHO's code: **ICD10-Z73.**

Many of us come to grief because we set unattainably high standards for ourselves, or sometimes the authorities set such targets. Joy comes when one realizes that in life we should try **to do our best; it need not be the best always.**

"Perfection shall be thy aim," said Jesus.

Further Reading

- Hans Selye. *Stress without Distress.* 1974.

CHAPTER 11

Matter of the Mind

Man is different from all other species on this planet in that his brain and all other organs could be influenced by his mind. The newer inventions in science have all been possible for man in this century and before, mainly because of his capacity to think. Although there has been a lot of thinking going on in medical circles about the role of the mind in psychological disorders, much needs to be done in the field of physical ailments. Recent data on the important role played by the human mind in the causation of major physical illnesses like heart attacks and cancer, have rekindled our interest in the intricacies of the working of the human mind vis-à-vis the human body. In the seventeenth century, William Harvey had clearly indicated that in all bodily afflictions there is a mental basis. Much work needs to be done in this direction. As there is no big money involved in this kind of research, the gold rush being in the field of epidemiology and interventions, the field did not, until very recently, attract good researchers. Funding agencies were also lukewarm to the research demands in this field.

The prestigious *Journal of the American Medical Association* in its recent issue (12 April 2000) has published a large study of the connection between life stresses and their role in the causation of coronary artery disease. This study is noteworthy in that it looked at the immediate and long-term effects of various emotional stressors that are a part of life in the modern rat race of the monetary economy. While there are many good studies published by the *British Medical Journal* during 2000–2003, before Dr Richard Smith retired as the editor, none of them have been as large as the study in the *JAMA* referred to earlier. Although significantly higher incidence of any disease in a group of human beings compared to another similar group does not definitely give a cause-effect relationship, the pointer in this instance is very significant.

Hostility, anger, frustration and bereavement come up on top among the negative emotions. Whereas previous studies have shown the good effects of positive emotions like love, compassion, social support, and job satisfaction, having control over one's situation, the present study has not looked at them in detail. The study clearly showed that many of these negative emotions acutely raised the blood pressure as also the heart rate and the breathing rate. It also indicated that chronic stress does take its toll on killer diseases. The role of emotions on chronic stable coronary disease, as also their role in precipitating the final assault either of a heart attack or sudden death, have been explored in detail. There is clear indication that emotions play a major role in the above situations.

So far so good. How do we change the emotions of the majority in society from the negative to the positive ones? This is the million-dollar question. While the study proclaims that behavioural changes, meditation, and stress management strategies do help, the authors have not done or reviewed any long term prospective study in this area, nor have they been able to fish out any randomized controlled study that has unequivocally shown that the methods mentioned above have really worked in real life situation. Here we need the help of the long-term longitudinal qualitative research of our ancient Ayurveda.

Our educational system hardly attempts to inculcate the values of good living and the fine art of living—live and let live. The basis of most depression (this has come up as the most important risk factor for both heart attacks and cancer) seems to be frustration in life. The latter results from man aiming his wants much higher than his needs. There is enough in this world for man's needs but not enough for man's greed. It is a curious observation that I have made over the last four decades that I have been interacting with patients that the incidence of depression is much higher among the well-to-do and the educated than the poor. If my observation is right, I have a hypothesis to offer. With affluence and so-called education of the present type, man becomes greedier and has more opportunities to get frustrated. Real happiness is in giving. If one learns to try and help others in need one gets busy and does not get time to think of the petty things that depress one.

Another area where we have a higher chance of depression is when our expectations are higher than what we are able to achieve. We are not taught by the educational system to be satisfied with what we are. When we try and project ourselves at a much higher level than our innate capacity and then fail to achieve what we want to, depression sets in. Jealousy is another of the negative feelings that triggers depression when one sees his opponent prospering. Life also becomes difficult if we expect too much from our near and dear ones. In the busy life of today, where one has to work hard to go up the ladder, one rarely finds time for others, more so the elders in the family, who are dependent on their progeny. Consequently, the elders who expect too much, get depressed. Ingratitude is another area where one could get depressed if he does not get due recognition for the favours he had bestowed on others. Money, rather the lack of it, is another potent cause of depression.

Quick-fix methods like drug treatment and psychotherapy might mitigate depression temporarily. However, the British study, as well as another Scandinavian study, have both clearly shown that depression, clinically obvious or occult, treated or otherwise, stood out as an independent risk for future heart attacks. This was also the experience of the doctors' study at the Johns Hopkins. This brings us to the point that it is better to primarily prevent depression in society. How do we do that?

The educational system should change from the present competitive ethos where one has to compete with another to the one where one competes with oneself for excellence. In the latter system there is no room for hatred and jealousy. In addition, value-based education could easily inculcate certain basic values in the child's impressionable mind. If only we could change the Macaulay type of education to our ancient Guru Kula type, one could avoid all the negative feelings getting into the child's head. Let our new schooling system not come in the way of the child's true education. Our only hope for the future is to bring up a whole new generation on this new educational ethos of excellence, camaraderie and co-operation, in place of competition, hatred and jealousy.

We have been having several quick fixes for our hapless victims of heart attacks and cancer through drugs, diet manipulation, and palliative surgical corrections. The scenario is no different in cancer therapy. We have spent too much time and money in copying the western model of curative medicine where, in fact, we have only been chasing a mirage. It is not what one eats that gets him into trouble, but it is what eats one that gets him into real trouble. That said, I must admit that the path is not strewn with rose petals even there. We have to work very hard at it to change the whole system what with all the vested interests trying to frustrate the efforts for their personal gains! But think we must in that direction. The journey of even hundred miles starts with the first step. Let us have the courage to take that first step.

> *Dimidium facti qui coepit,*
> *habet; sapere aude; incipe!*
>
> —Horace

(He who has begun his task has half done it. Have the courage to be wise. Begin!)

We cannot expect answers for many questions from any one. We will have to learn to think for ourselves. Indian Ayurvedic system had the wisdom to know that the mind sets the pace for all diseases, in this stanza:

> ***Khrodha, shokha, bhaya, aayaasa, virudhaanna bhojana,***
> ***Thaponnalaan, Katvaamla, kshaara,***
> ***lavana...raktha pitta prakopayeth.***

(Anger, intense worries (depression), fear, extreme exhaustion, sedentary life and many others things bring on all kinds of ailments.)

They also have given the remedy in the following stanza!

> ***Nithya hitha mitha aahaara sevi, sameekshakaari,***
> ***Dhata samaha sathyaapara, Khsamavaan,***
> ***Vishaye vasaakthaha, aapthopasevi,***
> ***Bhaveth aarogyam.***

(Eat food in moderation and that which pleases the mind, work very hard, avoid lies, hatred, and backbiting; have the courage to forgive even your enemy, always post-judge any issue, but to be healthy, in addition to all these, love everyone in this world as your dear and near ones)

A tall order, the skeptics would aver! True, it is a tall order, but not tall enough that ordinary mortals cannot reach. One only has to have the inclination and the right attitude based on sound value-based education to follow that dictum in life. This again is not possible if one has been brought up in the old style. I have been struggling to achieve that level of perfection but have failed time and again, but try again I do! It would be easy if we are brought up in that atmosphere right from the beginning. That is where my plea for change in our education set up for the new generation has some meaning.

The present day Yoga and meditation do precious little to make the practitioner tranquil, if the latter are not committed. The real yoga or meditation should aim at keeping the mind tranquil (*Chitta vritti nirodhaha yogaha*). Yoga should not be equated with aasanaas and simple meditation of closing the eyes and chanting some mantra. I feel that one could still do a lot by trying to be tranquil by living truthfully. It is in giving that you get. One could get peace of mind by trying to be of some use to someone else. That should be done with detachment. Indian philosophy gives a lot of food for thought in this direction. Materialism without a touch of spirituality would sink man into the valley of moral nihilism. Let us teach the next generation some values in life and hope for the best for the future of mankind.

Further Reading

- Strandberg TE, Salomaa VV, Naukkarinen VA, et al. Long-term mortality after 5-year multi-factorial primary prevention of cardiovascular diseases in middle aged men. *JAMA* 1991 Sep 4; 266(9): 1225–9.
- Linden W Stossel C and Maurice J Psycho-social interventions for patients with CAD. *Arch Intern Med.* 1996; 156: 745–752.

CHAPTER 12

On Doctoring

Medical Education

Should I tell how badly the present medical education needs drastic changes to be socially relevant? A recent UNIDO report shows that more than 80% of the world's population is not in touch with modern medicine of the type that we teach and practice. Their needs are only three:

- Clean drinking water
- Three square meals a day uncontaminated by human and/or animal excreta, and
- Economic empowerment to avoid the deadliest stress of not knowing where your next meal comes from.

All the improvement in human health has come from economic and sanitary improvement in human dwellings and not from the hi-tech medicine that is being touted as the panacea for all human ills. There is nothing like a pill for every ill. Medicine "cures rarely, comforts mostly, but consoles always."

To that end, we must restructure medical education to produce humane doctors who understand the agony and pain of suffering human beings to give succor to them. Present education throws up mostly good technicians that are good in "interventional medical techniques" but are bad, many a time, in dealing with suffering humanity.

The pinch is felt by many in the field, and one university, the Brisbane University in Australia, tries to pick medical students from among the graduates in humanities—arts, literature, music etc. Their experience has shown that this class of students would make better doctors; while the physics, chemistry and biology students make better technicians.

Two important areas need clarification to our students and doctors. One is that health of the public (public health) does not so much depend on medical quick-fix methods as it does on social changes in hygiene, food, and environmental factors. Let us keep these two on different pedestals, although both are needed for society. The other message is that life expectancy is only a statistical term denoting the number of years a newborn child could expect to live. It has nothing to do with life span at all. Many of us have this misconception that modern medicine has increased our life span. Far from it, very, very far. The truth is that modern medicine, if anything, has decreased our life span with many of the newer inventions and interventions!

Qualities of Head and Heart

A good doctor should be able to combine the qualities of the head and heart to be able to do most good to most people most of the time. On the bedside, even an illiterate patient very astutely studies the body language of the doctor. The patients and their relatives are always anxious when they are ill and they expect their doctor to be good, brave, efficient and kind—all at once. To be able to discharge one's duties as a good doctor, one should be able to combine the qualities of a strong head that could take difficult decisions even under very stressful situations, and the kindness of a large heart that has an insight into human suffering. The two key words that every young doctor should remember and revere are **imperturbability** and **equanimity.** Every word and action, including the mannerisms, is being watched carefully on the bedside by the sick individuals and, as such, they should be impeccable. Humility should be the watchword as **uncertainty** is the only **certainty** in medicine.

> Of the terrible doubt of appearances,
> Of the uncertainty after all-
> That we may be deluded...
>
> —*Walt Whitman*

Mistakes

Another area that needs clarification is in not telling our students in the college that doctors, like other human beings, are fallible. We are liable to make mistakes and that has to be made known to our patients, lest they should get the impression that doctors are Gods that never make mistakes. Now that we have given that impression and deified ourselves, any small mistake that we commit attracts lawsuits for compensation. This American disease is coming to other parts of the world in a big way, which would make medical care very expensive. Would you be surprised to know that in the USA more than 62% of upper middle class Americans cannot afford health insurance as the premia are too high, based on the star-performers' charges?

Medical education must aim at training the future doctors to accept the fact that human beings, doctors being human beings, make mistakes. The relatives and the patients would certainly understand and condone any genuine mistake done during a doctor discharging his/her duties. We must train students to develop to accept mistakes honestly and discuss the same plainly and in every detail with the patients and the relatives. Proper communication skills before and after treating a patient would enhance a better doctor-patient relationship, which has received a severe beating in the last couple of decades where technology has hijacked the time-honoured humane bedside medicine. Time was when doctors were very highly respected in society. Today, doctors are suspected as greedy, self-centered, and avaricious lot in society.

This has attracted the menace of consumerism into medicine. It is the medical profession that took medicine to the market place as a business, attracting the legal clause that medical care is a saleable commodity and the patient is a buyer. With this new equation today, judges perceive every suit filed against doctors seriously. To reverse this trend we must train our future doctors to be more humane and authentic.

Medical Science

The European universities accepted medicine as a scientific discipline around the beginning of the 12th century along with other natural sciences. However, the surgical specialties still remained outside the purview of the physicians; the former were still considered as skilled barber-surgeons. It was only in the 16th century with the advent of the Royal College of Surgeons in England that surgery was also included among medical sciences.

However, it is very important for a budding physician to realize that medicine is first and foremost an art, based on scientific principles. "Art" said Henry David Thoreau "is that which makes the man's day." The art of medicine is that which makes the patient's day – improves the quality of his life. It was Hippocrates who wrote, around the first century BC, that physicians "cure rarely, comfort mostly, but console always." This holds good even today. Most of what we do to our patients is to relieve pain and suffering. Whether doctors have the capacity to extend lifespan and to prevent death is a moot question.

Philosophically, death is the only certainty in life. Preventing death is against the natural laws, but alleviating pain, suffering and disability, should be our motto. To do that, doctors must learn "to do unto others what you would be done by". Empathy, where the doctor puts himself in the patient's shoes, should be the hallmark of the character development of any young doctor. It is only when we learn to empathize do we really become **placebo** doctors. Unfortunately, today's medical education produces doctors trained more as hi-tech technicians and not as holistic healers.

A healer needs a kind and a compassionate heart. Emotions do have a part to play in patient care; patient care being just **CARING** for the patient. Said Gautama Buddha "a doctor should look upon his patients just as the mother looks upon the child, her only child, bestowing all her love and attention on the child." Medical humanism should be a special subject for training doctors in medical schools. Technology and skill should only be added assets to a doctor but the core of every doctor should be qualities of love, compassion, caring and sharing.

The future of medical science, nay, other natural sciences, is in the capacity of these sciences to come together and understand one another, but not in getting further fragmented to the detriment of looking at the patient as a whole. The human body does not function in an organ-based isolation. The body works as a compact whole and not as a combination of its bits, working in different levels and directions. In addition, the human organism exists on this planet in symbiosis with all other living organisms of which there are billions and trillions around us.

Modern medicine followed natural sciences and their mathematical rules of linear systems. Although, physics, the king of sciences, left this narrow path a couple of decades ago after the advent of quantum physics, which has shown the futility of pursuing linear mathematical rules. Quantum physics has thrown up the existence of the human consciousness, which alone could gauge and assess the depths of this wonder, our Universe! Medical sciences did not follow suit; we continued our research efforts using reductionist methods.

Lately, a lot of well designed randomized studies both in the USA and UK have shown the vital role played by the human mind and emotions in bringing about the incidence and ravages of leading major killers like cancer, heart attack, stroke and even minor illness syndromes. These are mainly brought on by human emotions, rather than the conventional risk factors like cholesterol, etc. Scientists, both in the medical field and outside it, especially in quantum physics, have realized that one cannot work and understand the workings of this universe, man included, without the help of the human mind.

Where is the mind? Never mind! This simple answer would no longer hold water. The human mind is not an organ-based cytopathological structure; it is in the realm of the sub-atomic quantum field in every single human body cell, of which there are one hundred thousand billion in all. Werner Heisenberg's **Uncertainty Principle** and Erwin Schrödinger's **Cat Hypothesis** have shown, very clearly, that excluding human mind would not solve problems. I hope thinking people would now believe that the time has come to take another look at the medical education doled out in our schools which, probably, would bring out excellent medical technicians skilled in interventions, but do not bring out humane healers.

Continuing Professional Development

"Half of what man knows today would be proved wrong in five years' time, but the problem with mankind is that they would not know which half it is", wrote Cicero, the great Roman thinker. This is truer in medicine where, on an average, 35,000 new publications come out every month in the innumerable biomedical journals mushrooming all over. One needs to keep in touch to be able to deliver the correct line of management every time a patient seeks advice. Mandatory re-certification is being thought of, but it is imperative that every doctor keeps himself up-to-date with his specialty always, in addition to self-learning from one's mistakes. The latter is very precious empirical experience that helps in patient care.

Research

Research is an integral part of teaching. The greatest research in the past has been the observational research of our ancestors. Although we have produced a surfeit of research data with more than 35,000 research papers coming out every month in the innumerable biomedical journals, a recent audit showed that less than 1% of it is making any mark in advancing human wisdom. Future research must concentrate on the need-based, locally relevant, problem solving questions rather than replicating what the advanced West does, to publish or perish. Repetitive research does not widen our horizon. There are innumerable myths in medicine, which need to be demolished. The quicker we do it the better for the suffering humanity.

**Knowledge advances NOT by repeating known facts,
But by refuting false dogmas.**

—*Karl Popper*

A recent UNIDO report showed how modern hi-tech medicine did not reach the majority of suffering human beings in the world, who still lack the basic amenities of life like clean water, three square meals a day and a healthy environment to live in. Poverty still is the largest risk factor for disease. In addition, it is a double-edged sword. While poverty brings on more illness, the resulting illness deprives the hapless victim of his earning capacity. It thus cuts both ways. Economic empowerment of the masses and alleviation of poverty are as vital to reduce the disease load in society, as it is to palliate the existing diseases.

As modern medicine quick fixes are absolutely necessary in emergency situations, many of the chronic illnesses and minor illness syndromes either do not benefit from the top-heavy modern medical establishment, or could do well with very inexpensive but effective alternative systems of medicine, of which there are many in our country. Whereas it is mandatory that we teach our students the usefulness and the existence of these systems as also the public dependence on them, we must work fast to sift the wheat from the chaff in those complementary systems, by using the touchstone of modern scientific methodology. Here again, having a holier-than-thou approach has been counterproductive. We should be able to take our holistic approach forwards with the help of the other systems and not by having an ostrich-like attitude in condemning the latter.

I wish all the young entrants into the noble profession, God speed and good luck. May they be enthused to commit themselves to public health, the health of the public. Let them be very clear in their mind that the profession of medicine is not for making money primarily, although money would automatically come, but to keep society as healthy as is humanly possible. I hope the budding physicians would have the continued patronage and support of their teachers and parents in their journey to help society.

> **To handle yourself use your head,**
> **To handle others, use your heart.**
>
> —Anon

Further Reading

- Reynolds R, Stone J. *On Doctoring.* 1991. Simon and Schuster, New York.
- Pickering WG. Does medical treatment mean patient benefit? *Lancet* 1996;347: 379–80.

CHAPTER 13

Future Medicare System

> Men are disturbed not by things which happen,
> but by the opinions about the things.
>
> —*Epictetus;* First Century Greek Philosopher

Modern medicine has become prohibitively expensive. It is going to be still more so with newer technology invading medical diagnosis and management more and more. Most of these technologies have not been audited and some of those that were inadvertently audited did not live up to the expectations of their promoters and, in some instances, have even caused more harm than good. It is estimated that around 80% of the world population have not been availing the modern medical facilities! Around half of the rest who have even free access to modern medicine would prefer to have an alternative system, if available, even in the industrialized West. The reasons for the disillusionment are protean, but the lack of medical humanism is one of the foremost.

Oregon state in the USA realized, to its dismay, that one bone marrow transplant in a terminally ill cancer child would cost as much to the taxpayer as looking after the health needs of one thousand pregnant women through pregnancy and delivery, as also the health needs of the baby for the first year of life. Recently, they enacted the Oregon Law that bans bone marrow transplants for terminally ill cancer children at the taxpayer's cost. This did create trouble in the beginning but, eventually, many other states have followed suit. This could give one an idea of the magnitude of the financial load of covering every citizen with all the technology available, even in the rich nations. Most of these techniques only make life *appear longer* making the patient a slightly better cripple.

Let us not bother to look at the scenario in the poorer countries for the purposes of this chapter. Suffice it to quote the recent WHO document (WHO 2002) that shows that if the people of the poorer nations were to get clean drinking water, it would bring down two million deaths per year and prevent half a billion serious illnesses. Obviously, our priorities are skewed very badly. The western pharmaceutical industry, however, is trying to push costly, many times unproven, drugs and technology into the third world, where even today the common man does not have access to clean drinking water, three meals a day with food uncontaminated by human and/or animal excreta, and a toilet to avoid the deadly hookworm infestation of children!

Need for a New Paradigm in Medical Care

Robust circumstantial evidence goes to show that 80% of the world population that does not have access to modern medicine lives using their intuition in times of need and get benefits from many other time-tested alternative systems of medicine, many of them being much more ancient compared to modern medical wisdom. One of them, the Indian system of *Ayurveda,* is much more ancient, having survived the discouragement in the recent past even in India. We now have unequivocal data to show that Ayurveda is the mother of most other systems, notably the modern medical system. Present day modern medicine originated in the Nile Valley five thousand years ago as sorcery, witchcraft, magic and mumbo-jumbo. In the present day, "much of the news and advertisements of health education with which we are bombarded are designed to heighten our worries, not soothe them; many drug companies play upon our tendencies toward hypochondriasis," Wrote Herbert Benson in his celebrated book *Timeless Healing.*

In its onward journey through Arabia and then Greece, modern medicine came under the spell of Ayurveda taken to Greece by the army of Alexander the Great. There are two authentic works to support this hypothesis. *India in Greece* is an excellent treatise written by a great Greek scholar, E Pococke, who lived in India for years. He wrote this book in 1832 AD. Another authoritative book is the one on *Ancient Indian Medicine* written in 1936 by Late Prof P Kutumbiah, MD, FRCP, who served as the Professor of Medicine both, in Vellore and, later, at the Madras Medical College.

This apart, the popular belief about the eradication of the only scourge of mankind, smallpox, needs a major change to get at the truth. Dr TZ Holwell, FRS, was a Fellow of the London Royal College of Physicians. He spent twenty years in "The Bengal Province" of the Raj to study the Indian system of vaccination and its effect in preventing small pox. After twenty years of prospective controlled studies, he concluded, in his report to the Royal College, submitted in the year 1767 AD, that the Indian system of vaccination, which existed for "times out of mind," with a type of attenuated small pox virus, was ninety per cent effective in preventing small pox deaths and had very little side effects. This report, in its original shape, is still available in the archives of the College library. It cannot be photostatted but is in the Internet as a Revised Version. Surprisingly, it survived the great fire in the library some years later. Holwell favoured permitting the anecdotal experience of Edward Jenner to be used freely in view of the Indian experience of antiquity! He pleaded with the President and Fellows of the Royal College to recommend to the King the free use of Jenner's unproven method in view of his solid proof from Indian vaccination system. The rest is history known to all.

Suggested New Classification of Diseases

To understand the new paradigm one needs to classify human diseases based on the treatment needs thus:

- Emergency medicine — 10% of the sick population
- Minor illness syndromes — 35% ibid
- Doctor-Thinks-You-Have-a-Disease — 15% ibid
- Patient-Thinks-He-has-a-Disease — 10% ibid
- Neoplasias — 10% ibid
- Chronic degenerative diseases — 10% ibid
- Iatrogenic diseases — 10% ibid

Classified like this, most of the diseases, where modern hi-tech medicine, with all the glittering array of diagnostic tools, the expensive interventions and drugs are of utmost need, fall into the first category of emergency diseases. The new specialty of emergency medicine in the west is the most welcome timely step in the right direction. Rather, it heralds the need for the paradigm shift, referred to elsewhere. It is here that the advances of modern medicine could make a dent in improving the lot of the suffering humanity and, possibly, also in preventing avoidable deaths. In the emergency set-up, even unproven technology could be justifiably used in extreme situations.

Time has come for a proper audit of the present use of hi-tech medicine under all the illness situations classified above. I strongly feel that in non-emergency situations we need not (possibly, should not) resort to hi-tech modern medical help. We could easily put together an inexpensive method of managing most of those 90% illnesses using a judicious mix of the best in many useful alternative systems of medical care. Rarely, in some of those situations, like the neoplasias, modern medicine could be used in conjunction with scientifically tested alternatives, to reduce the cost and the intolerable side effects of chemotherapy and radiation. The latter two have not shown themselves in very good light so far.

Many of the newer, yet to be tested, but much hyped, chemotherapeutics are prohibitively expensive for the poor. These methods of cancer management have not made a significant dent in total cancer deaths. Cancer deaths have still to level off before showing a tendency to come down. This could be contested using statistical methods known to modern researchers, though.

There are excellent remedies for the control and/or prevention of the major class of minor illness syndromes that cause the largest sick absenteeism in productive fields everyday, in *Ayurveda* as well as other alternative systems. Some of them have been tested by the modern medical methods already. The powerful anti-viral properties of Indian spices, mainly garlic, ginger, and pepper have been studied in the leading western laboratories. More than all that is the thrust in Ayurveda of methods to keep the healthy well. These health-promotive strategies are the backbone of *Ayurveda*.

Swasthasya swastha rakshitham.
(Keep the well healthy)

This is the most important slogan in that system and there are many methods of health-promotion based on life style changes, food habits, exercise, yoga, meditation (making the mind tranquil), and also certain herbal remedies to slow the ageing process. Unfortunately, quacks and unqualified people have brought disrepute to most of those systems. It is because those methods have not been scientifically evaluated before being let loose on the gullible public. This must stop forthwith!

The reader could be surprised to know that the ancient school of medicine of Shushruta needed a much longer period of training to be a doctor than most modern medical schools today. The students studied human anatomy in much greater detail for much longer time to achieve perfection! All these need to be looked into before we jump on the new bandwagon of other systems. What I am advocating is not too many systems to be used concurrently. The best brains in the various systems will have to put their heads together to evolve a new system, the **complementary system of medical care,** that has a scientifically judicious mix of the best in all those systems along with the emergency hi-tech care for a holistic medical care delivery system that could economically do most good to most people most of the time.

There was an audit of the effect of modern medicine in the USA about two decades ago. Whereas **59%** of the improvement in human health and fall in disease incidence there could be attributed to improvement in sanitation, improved nutrition, better education, decent housing, economic empowerment of the masses, and healthier life style avoiding tobacco and alcohol, **only 3.4%** of the change could be due to modern medical claptrap! One needs to repeat this in many other countries to get a better picture that might motivate even the skeptics to agree to the paradigm shift.

Surprisingly, even in the emergency set up, although I feel that the latter definitely needs hi-tech, a comparative study of the per capita deaths of the wounded soldiers in the Vietnam and Falklands wars did show that it was marginally better in Falklands compared to Vietnam. While the American soldiers in Vietnam had the best base hospital in the nearby Saigon, the British did not have such luxury in the South American war theatre. Many a time the wounded soldiers in Falklands were left to be tended by the forces of Nature, before being attended to and, that too, not in a sophisticated hi-tech modern base hospital. One of the explanations for this disparity could be that we have been interfering with Nature's methods of dealing with human injury with the help of the sympathetic system evolved to protect the hunter-gatherer forefather of man from the most important danger those days: predation!

Complementary Medical Care Delivery System

The idea of mooting this strategy is to stimulate people to think about this possibility to make medical care available to all the people of the world, rich and poor, that is not only equally effective but cost effective as well. **We must take care to see that the new system is put in place after due care to see that untested, unproven, and potentially dangerous methods do not get included.** The scientific methods and agencies overseeing this stupendous task must not only be highly competent, but should be equally authentic. We hear of the fraud in medical research in modern medicine almost daily, to be brushed aside lightly. With that background in view, the people at the helm of affairs must have a proven track record.

There would be great opposition from the all-powerful drug and technology lobbies that literally run medical education in the west these days. They start brainwashing future doctors from day one at medical school, only to stop at their graves! It is heartening to know, though, that there are very good people even in those areas, but they are like an occasional oasis in vast desert sand and are an endangered species, indeed. We should be able to get their help in this humanitarian venture.

With the present worldwide communication facilities the task of bringing the best people together need not be difficult. Well meaning people in the modern medical field should take the lead to bring respectability to this effort. We need to do a lot of education of the common man and the media to accept this line of thinking in the midst of powerful and rich medical claptrap. The latter has a vested interest in keeping the system as it is. **The present hi-tech medical care delivery system is a big business. This is the very reason why medicine has lost its heart today**. The time-honored doctor patient relationship is replaced by the doctor being viewed as the seller and the patient the buyer of medical technology, bringing in its wake the consumer movement into medicine. The crux of the medical scenario is the trust that the patient has in his/her doctor that provokes the immune system to heal the sick. Healing is a much larger concept than the concept of "curing" used commonly by doctors. Doctors only dress the wound; the immune system heals it. Let us bring back the patient confidence in his/her doctor back into the medical arena for the common good, before it is lost for ever.

No man, no author, not even the greatest, ever provides the last word on anything. Men are vain authorities who can resolve nothing. (II, 13)

—*Michel de Montaigne*

Further Reading

- Robin ED. Death by Pulmonary Artery Flow Directed catheter. Time for a moratorium. *Chest* 1987; 92: 727–729
- Steven Milloy. *Science without Sense*, 1997. Cato Institute, Washington
- *New Scientist,* 17th September 1994, page 23

- *Ancient Indian Medicine*, Kutumbiah P. Oxford University Press
- Benson H. *Timeless Healing*. 1996 Simon and Shuster, Sydney
- Hegde BM. Vaccination in India, *JAPI* 1998; 46: 472–473
- Hegde BM. Are We Barking up the wrong tree? *The Cardiologist* 2000:Vol. 3, No. 4:1–3
- Coleman V. The betrayal of Trust, *European Med J*. 1994; :4
- Editorial. Flight from Science. *BMJ* 1980; : 1–2
- Editorial. Drug company influence on medical education in the USA. *Lancet* 2000; 356: 781
- Austin JA. Why patients use alternative medicines? *JAMA* 1998; 279: 1548-53
- Weil A. The significance of integrative medicine for the future of medical education. *Am J Med* 2000; 108: 441–443
- Smith GD, and Ebrahim S. Data Dredging, bias, or confounding. *BMJ* 2002; 325: 1437–1438
- Bernardi L, Bandinelli G, Cencetti S, et al. Effect of rosary prayer and yoga mantras on autonomic cardiovascular rhythms: Comparative study. *BMJ*; 2001; 323: 1446–1449

CHAPTER 14

Medical Philosophy

No great discovery was ever made in science except by one who lifted his nose above the grindstone of details and ventured on to more comprehensive vision.
—*Albert Einstein*

I wonder, at times, in real life situations, if we have lost our sense of direction in modern medicine, by relying solely on reductionist science. We have enough evidence to show that this kind of logic does not work in any dynamic system, least of all in the human being, which is much more than the organs that we are trying to "fix." Each time we feel that some "things" have gone wrong with the human organs; we try and "do" something, until the patient gets better or he dies. Death of a patient makes us feel, for a while, that we could be inadequate, possibly fallible, and could be wrong in our approach to the whole gamut of curing, while we should have been healing, instead. The essence of medical teaching these days seems to be, a "do it" and "fix it" attitude. Deep down, this is driven by the technological onslaught into this humane calling, the healing art.

"Art" is defined by Henry David Thoreau as "that which makes a man's day." Healing art is that which makes the patient's day. The doctor-patient relationship is akin to any other archetypal human behavior, like that of the mother-child or husband-wife relationship. What does that mean in practical terms? Every man brings with him to this world that innate quality of human interaction, which, basically, governs his personality. In every doctor there is the wounded patient and the healer, as there is in every patient an innate capacity to be a healer as well as a wounded sufferer. This is an ancient mythological concept, if you wish. Maharani was both the giver and healer of smallpox, in Indian mythology. In Babylon, there was the story of the dog-Goddess with two names, "as Gulag she was death, and as Labarum a healer."

Unfortunately, modern medicine rarely takes a serious note of the "healer" in the patient, adopting mostly a paternalistic attitude "to cure," which many a time fails to work or even could work against the patient (iatrogenic disease). **The greatest discovery of the twentieth century has been the discovery of man's ignorance.** However, this does not seem to have percolated to reductionist science and medicine in a significant way. The word `doctor' is derived from the etymological root "to docere," meaning "to teach." A good teacher is one "who knows not, and knows, he knows not." Together with his student, curiosity should compel him to ponder over the unknown. This is a great quality, which tries to help the student deliver the goods. Education is derived from the Greek root (e=out, ducere=to bring out *the baby)*. It is the student who ultimately has to bring out the child. On the same analogy, it is the patient who has to heal himself, awakening his `inner doctor'—the immune system.

Lewis Thomas, the former President of the Sloane Kettering Cancer Institute, in New York once wrote, "Instead of always emphasizing what we actually know in science, it would be enormously fruitful to focus alternatively on what we do not know. For it is here that the wonders lie. To know is the domain that is safe, where risk taking is no longer necessary. To dwell in it forever is not only to never advance, it is also to promote a deceptive and false view of ourselves as knowing more than we do, of being more powerful than we really are."

The above idea clearly diagnoses the cancer that is eating into modern medicine and its reductionist scientific basis. The latter, however, is gradually dying a natural death, weighed down by specialization and sub-specialization. There, in the distant horizon, is the rising of the new sun—the science of CHAOS and non-linear mathematics. We cannot be oblivious to this fact, as medicine controls the lives of millions of people who are ill, or imagine they are ill, at any given point in time. We need a new philosophy of holism in medicine, in the true sense of the word.

If one observes human growth on this planet, one notices a ceaseless transformation of his intellect from the cave-dwelling forefathers' time of the "me" concept to the "other than me" reality. In this continuum man has grown from the "single me" to a group, then to a village, to a city, to a nation, and now to the whole universe! I am happy that it is the Indian thought that has been always ahead of others in this field. The Vedic wisdom of **Vasudai Eva Kutumbikam** (this whole world is but one family) shows that our ancestors could think clearly much ahead of their times. We urgently need such visionaries, who dare to lift medicine from the bottomless pit dug up by technology-money-business attitude.

Why does one get any disease? It is a million-dollar question! Charles Sherrington, the famous physiologist, in the year 1899, at the age of forty-two, when he was appointed professor of physiology at the Liverpool University, said in his acceptance speech:

The question "why" can never be answered by positive science. The latter can, at best, answer the question "how" or "how much" but never the question "why." A physiologist could say how the heart contracts, but never say why the heart contracts; he could define death, but will never be able to define life. Ratio rei is, therefore, not reason why! How true?

The question "why" could only be answered in teleology, but never in biology. Let us now examine the new concept in teleology. The Universal consciousness would want this world to go on uninterrupted, or at least, without much damage to its components. Naturally, all bad people, who could be a nuisance to society will, eventually, have to be eliminated or, at least, immobilized, to avoid unnecessary trouble for the good people in the world. People who are angry, jealous, proud, hostile, and greedy are a menace to society. Recent studies have thrown up every one of the above devils to be important risk factors for all the dangerous and fatal degenerative illnesses.

Dawson Churchill writes:

"From the global perspective it may be very valuable that such an individual be unhealthy. This limits his scope of working mischief! If he were well, his ability to project these destructive emotions into disruptive action would be enhanced. Illness may thus be something of a planetary defense mechanism, a reaction against baneful inner states, which human beings have nurtured within themselves."

Although I may not agree with his views in toto, they look very logical and holistic. **This is in fact the global wellness concept that I have been developing over the years. Nothing in this universe could be viewed in isolation.** This concept tries to marry biology to teleology, answering both the questions "why" and "how".

On the other side is the enormous "progress" that we have made in the medical technological field. We live in an age of heart transplants, artificial hearts and kidneys, genetic engineering, and even cloning. Daily we wage surgical and chemical warfare on diseases and the bill for it all is skyrocketing. Star-performers in the field are attracting all the limelight; and the price tags keep going up keeping pace with those stars' charges. Writing an editorial in the *New England Journal of Medicine,* Professor Krumholtz, a leading cardiologist at Yale University, wrote about the business going on in the field of the most expensive of interventions, the bypassing of the coronary heart vessels by surgery. He felt that bypass surgery is done more often to fill the coffers of hospitals and surgeons, rather than to help patients. Many studies in this field are being twisted, using all sorts of statistics, to show benefit to the patient, while in essence, the procedures are only helping the doctors and the industry. Corporate business houses are jumping into the arena of "hospital industry" in the fond hope of making large profits, without much headache from labour unions or raw material suppliers. This goes against all canons of medical ethics, if there are any left, of Hippocrates: *"never try to make money in the sick room."* Did he say that you should do free service? Far from it, very far! What he meant was that medicine is a calling, which is very noble, and should never be debased to that of a moneymaking business.

Running parallel to this development is the burgeoning undercurrent of mistrust and loss of faith in the medical profession, noticed by the galloping law suits against doctors in the West, which is, sadly, making a foray into our country as well. This doctor-distrust would make medicine very expensive, in that every doctor, under all circumstances, would want to use every available technological test, to allay his own anxiety, to protect himself against a future potential threat of legal action. This is where we stand today.

With this background, it is time for us to take another look at what we are doing in modern medicine; the latter being based mainly on the old Newtonian physics and linear mathematics. In this century, beginning with Einstein's theory of special effects in 1905, and later his *Theory of Relativity,* followed by further developments in quantum physics of time, space, energy, and matter, the scientific world started coming nearer to the ancient wisdom of the East, which looks at this world as a whole, including the observer's consciousness. Werner Heisenberg's *Uncertainty Principle* ultimately brought modern science very close to Adi Shankara's philosophy of the uncertainty principle of matter, energy, and the *Maya.*

Technological, market-force driven, modern medicine has to change, to keep pace with man's wisdom, driving him slowly towards the *Ultimate Truth*. "Modern Medicine", said Prince Charles, heir to the British Throne, *"with all its breathtaking progress, is like the Tower of Pisa, slightly off balance."* I could not agree more! Doctors, like others in all walks of life, should have their **swadharma (societal obligations).** The following Indian oath of the physician is worth noting in this context.

- You must be chaste and abstemious, speak the truth, and not eat meat.
- Care for the good of all living beings; devote yourself to the healing of the sick even if your life were lost by your work.
- Do the sick no harm; not, even in thought, seek another's wife or goods; be simply clothed and drink no intoxicant; speak clearly, gently, truly, and properly; consider time and place; always seek to grow in knowledge.
- Treat women except their men be present; never take a gift from women without her husband's consent.
- When the physician enters a house accompanied by a man suitable to introduce him there, he must pay attention to all the rules of behavior in dress, deportment, and attitude.
- Once with his patient, he must in word and thought attend to anything but his patient's case and what concerns it. What happens in the house must not be mentioned outside, nor must he speak of possible death to his patients, if such a speech is liable to injure him or anyone else.
- In the face of Gods and man you can take upon yourself these vows; may all the Gods aid you if you abide thereby; otherwise may all the Gods and the sacra, before which we stand, be against you;

And the pupil should consent to this, saying,

"So be it."

FURTHER READING

- Hippisley Cox J, Pringle M, and Feilding K. Depression as a risk factor for ischaemic heart disease in men. *BMJ* 1998; 316: 1714–19.
- Whiteman MC, Fowkes FGR, and Deary IJ: Hostility and the Heart. (Editorial). *BMJ* 1997;315:379–80.
- Hegde BM. Medical Humanism. *Proc Roy Coll Phy (Edin.)* 1997;27:65–67.
- Church D, Sherr A (Ed.) *The Heart of the Healer*. Signet Books, Canada 1987.
- Hegde BM. Consumerism in Medicine. *J Ind Med Assn*. 1996;94:154–155.

CHAPTER 15

Primum Non Nocere
(First, Do No Harm)

A thing is not necessarily true because a man dies for it.

—Oscar Wilde (1854–1900) in *Sebastian Melmoth* (1904 Ed)

It is time to ask the question whether Hippocrates was right in proclaiming the above dictum for all future followers of his craft? The more I learn about our profession the less faith I have in the truth of the Hippocratic Oath. People are after fame, mystery, falsehood, and false prestige and, of course, money. I can understand the latter but why the former? Life has taught me that it is the former that facilitates the latter. The man, who does genuine hard work, using his own special powers of thinking and comes up with an innovative idea rarely, if ever, gets his due credit. It is the crafty ones that could steal that wisdom and use it to perform "miracles," that get the limelight and all that goes with it. It is not the one whose genius discovers something that gets the limelight but the one who somehow or the other convinces the world about it gets all the benefits. That is life! The story keeps repeating itself again and again. May be that is why the intellectual property right has come in!

Here is the true story behind the **"*first*" heart transplant** that the world has come to believe in. Time was when South Africa, with its despicable apartheid policy, was getting totally isolated in the international community; it needed to achieve something that the world could be proud of. It is a fact that South Africa had one of the best medical care delivery systems in the world at that time coupled with full time teachers doing excellent basic research in the medical school. To cap it, they did not have much consumer awareness and ethical committees' hindrance for any kind of research. That was the time that a young man, Christian Barnard, came back after training in cardiac surgery both in the UK and the USA to join a team of researchers. He was itching to make it big and get into the limelight at any cost. In the words of one of his close associates, he was "ruthless, egocentric, hardworking, clever, ambitious, brash, and downright arrogant."

One example of his qualities of head and heart manifesting could be shown in the following anecdote. When a Russian surgeon reported an operation where he had transplanted an extra head to a dog, Barnard repeated that feat with great difficulty to show that "he could do anything that anyone else did." He was very proud of his grotesque operation with the dog having two heads and got it widely publicized! Barnard's arrogance was responsible for the "truly" first transplant patient paying for the operation with his own life. After the heart transplant operation Barnard irradiated his patient with whole body radiation to suppress the immune rejection, while it was an established practice with kidney transplants not to have total body irradiation, in 1967. Barnard deliberately rejected that practice to show that his patient's graft rejection was negligible. He was right that the graft did not get rejected but, the patient died of severe infection in both his lungs due to iatrogenic (doctor induced) immune deficiency.

It was 3rd December 1967 at the Groote Schuur Hospital, South Africa, where a young female accident victim was admitted for observation. The following day the doctors "***decided***" that she had no chance of survival at all. Christian Barnard was impatiently waiting to immediately grab the opportunity to do his ***"truly" first*** heart transplant operation on a middle-aged man suffering from terminal heart failure. The heart of the young lady was still beating normally when removed to be used for the man! Unfortunately for all concerned, the patient died in a few days' time with massive bilateral pneumonia. This was never reported in the media.

Two weeks later another golden opportunity came looking for Barnard. A young white man was admitted after having gone swimming, and was brought to the hospital unconscious. He had a subarachnoid haemorrhage. He was not making any progress. Dr (now Sir) Raymond Hoffenberg was the physician in charge. Pressure was being brought upon Sir Raymond to declare the young man brain dead, but he was not in fact brain dead at all. Even the definition of brain death that existed then looks so flawed today that most of the declared brain dead donors could well have lived on for many years with normal life! Even the present definition of brain death is far from satisfactory. Barnard was later to be acclaimed as the most heroic of surgeons in the eyes of the public. He also earned tons of money. Of course, the heroes in the game were the hapless accident victims and the poor recipients.

The medical wisdom at that time was that transplants could survive only with beating hearts and not cadaver hearts. So Barnard was looking for beating hearts all over the place. Poor patients admitted at that time in South Africa must have been really unlucky. In the company of a man with a hammer who wants to use it badly everything would look like a nail needing hammering. Every accident victim was a potential donor for Barnard. Sir Raymond Hoffbenberg was to be deported under the "suppression of communism" act of South Africa the following day. Early in the morning he was somehow or other "forced" (I would not know for certain what went through his mind at that time, although he claimed later that most of the patient's reflexes were unelicitable by the time he decided to declare her brain dead, but her heart was still healthy and beating) to sign a declaration that the accident victim was brain dead. Before that the Head of surgery was very unhappy with Sir Raymond. "What sort of a heart are you going to give us eventually?" he once asked angrily.

Soon the whole hospital was electrified. Everyone was excited, as they were to make history of sorts! Dr Philip Blaiberg, a South African dentist, was in the hospital with intractable heart failure. He received this accident victim's heart "successfully". **This was proclaimed to the world as the FIRST heart transplant.** Another! indeed! Blaiberg lived for 18 months. The media was told that he lived a near normal life. He is said to have indulged in sexual intercourse with his wife. He was shown to be swimming in the sea to prove to the world that heart transplants are very useful. The fact is that Blaiberg was almost as ill as he was before the operation. **The whole publicity was a hoax**. He was taken to the sea in a "hi-tech ambulance" and lowered to the level of the water by a team of doctors and nurses. The latter stood away for a fraction of a second for the photographers to click. Blaiberg was immediately lifted up before he went under the waves. As far as the sexual act was concerned, I feel the press did not press for the photographs, if it ever happened! The syndicated photograph of Blaiberg swimming in the sea made so many cardiac surgeons all over the world so jealous that in one year in 1968, one hundred and seven "copycat" operations were done in 24 countries by sixty-four surgical teams, some of them with disastrous consequences.

One such operation was done that year in the then Bombay City in India also. The operation was successful but the patient, of course, died almost at the end of the operation. Dr. Sen was a very good man and did not believe in false publicity. Prof Sen was a great researcher, having had many innovative procedures to his credit. He openly told the press that the patient died immediately after the operation. A less ethical doctor in his place would have told a lie and kept the patient artificially breathing for sometime at least.

On the 30th December 1967, the *South African Medical Journal* brought out a special issue in commemoration of Barnard's feat with many articles and an editorial on heart transplantation, making Christian Barnard a cult figure. Basically a showman, Barnard "indulged in an impetuous, flamboyant, global lap of honor." Once again the Government of South Africa sent him on a world tour with his wife and some of his teammates for other big television shows around the world. Money and fame followed soon after.

To give you an idea of how these great feats are accomplished at the cost of the poor patients and then given wide publicity, I shall quote another event in Barnard's life that will show the man in his true colour. *Time* magazine was to honour the first man who initiated the artificial heart. An American showman wanted to grab that honor, but Michael DeBakey, a Lebanese-born American, had been the father of artificial hearts, having devised it first. To outwit DeBakey this actor surgeon got a letter written by Christian Barnard to him antedated six months earlier, congratulating him for inventing the artificial heart, thus making sure that *Time* magazine gave equal, if not better, credit to him! Arrogant as he was Barnard could not keep this secret. He told his friends in his department about it. He also told his associates that he did this favour because he expected the other gentleman to reciprocate similar favours.

The story of Werner Forssmann's story is still more pathetic. He was the first to insert a catheter into his own heart while he was still a trainee surgeon. This was criticized severely. While some colleagues, claiming priority accused him of plagiarism, others dismissed his feat as irresponsible. He did not get his credit for a long time until one day in the year 1956 he was awarded the Nobel Prize when he was practicing surgery in a small village for his living, forgotten by the world. When informed by the press, Forssmann is reported to have exclaimed: "I feel like a village parson who has just learned that he has been made the bishop!" His boss, the "greatest" German surgeon in the 20s, Herr *Geheimrat* Sauerbruch, at the Charite in 1929 wanted the credit for himself! When Forssmann went to see Sauerbruch at the Charite the office manager is said to have rebuked him by saying that: "In this hospital one does not present himself to the Herr *Geheimrat, one waits to be summoned...!"*

I could give you another example of frauds that the so-called great people commit. DeBakey, the innovative surgeon, was operating on a middle-aged patient trying to replace his badly damaged aortic valve. When he went in he found that the valve was badly calcified, and the mouths of the coronary arteries were almost closed up. He wondered as to how he could make this man live after the valve replacement without good blood supply to his heart muscle. Here, he tried his new idea successfully. He had been toying with the idea of bypassing a blocked coronary artery with leg veins. He did not venture into that area, as he was not convinced that it was a very good physiological solution to the problem! He must have been a brilliant man. His doubts have now been proven to be well-founded. However, with the patient on the table he had to do something on the spot, however bad it could be in the long run. Pressed to the wall, he harvested the saphenous vein of the patient from the leg and reversed it to make a "jump-graft" from the proximal aorta to the distal portion of the patient's coronaries—**the first bypass surgery in a patient (1963).**

The patient did very well, but, DeBakey did not tell the world what he did, as he wanted to study what would happen to the patient in the long run— the true scientific way. To his bad luck, another surgeon did a successful copycat bypass surgery in 1967 learning the technique from Fulvero. This was reported in the same year making it the first operation of that kind. ***It was only in 1968, after five years' observations, did DeBakey tell the world about the bypass surgery and showed that a patient could live that long, as it was not known at that time.*** This is true science. Similar stories abound in other countries, including India. Unfortunately, it is the first category of copycats that get all the media publicity. It is true all over the world. If you try to get to the bottom of medical history, most celebrated events are only medical claptrap.

In the bargain, the man who struggled to discover the methods of heart transplant and many other innovative methods in cardiac surgery, Norman Shumway, the chief of cardiac surgery at Stanford, was forgotten. He quietly worked to perfect the technique that Barnard learnt from him and waited until basic scientific advances were made, so he could perform safer human transplants. He waited until cadaver hearts could be successfully transplanted, as he did not want to "kill" the donor to harvest a beating heart. Since then he probably has had the largest number of successful heart transplants done without fanfare and media publicity. The one time Barnard was dumbfounded in his rhetoric was when the ITV interviewer, the famous David Frost, confronted him with two uncomfortable questions. One: "Did you kill the donor for Blaiberg to get publicity for yourself?" And the other: "Did you not ride piggyback on your mentor Norman Shumway and steal his secrets?"

Barnard did wriggle out by saying that he did not get the secrets from Norman, but from an article that the father of British cardiac surgery, Sir Russel Brock, wrote about the feasibility of heart transplants years ago. For the other question he said that the definition of brain death at that time allowed him to take the beating heart. So much for probity in medical research. If they are genuine they do not need publicity. My suggestion to medical students is not to believe every printed word as gospel truth. There is a lot that does not get to the textbooks for obvious reasons. **Truth is the first casualty in a world that runs on money and false glamour. Falsehood and mystery would drag millions by the nose. Truth, on the contrary, can influence only a score of people in a century. This was the opinion of Aristotle.**

> **Tis strange-but true; for truth is always strange;**
> **Stranger than fiction...**
>
> —Lord Byron (1788–1824): in *Don Juan* 1819–1824

FURTHER READING

- Sir Raymond Hoffenberg. Christian Berbard and his first transplant—on concepts of death. *BMJ* 2001; 323: 1478–1480

- Werner Forssmann. *Experiments on Myself.* 1974. Saint Martin's Press, New York. (Originally published in Germany in 1972 translated by Hillary Davies)

CHAPTER 16

Primary Health Care

What our age lacks is not reflection but passion.

—Soren Kierkegaard

Health is the first casualty in our villages and also in bigger cities. Whereas the latter have many large and small hospitals, both in public and private sectors, vying with one another for patients, in addition to some really five-star hospitals for the upper income group, our villages, of which there are more than six hundred thousand, lack proper medical facilities, not to speak of any health facilities worth their name. Even the large cities have dismal health preserving facilities!

You may think I am splitting hair here. Far from it. The modern medical set ups, including the teaching institutions, indirectly stress on quick fixes for illnesses and do not really stress the need to preserve health. One could argue that the preventive health practices of the western variety, with their emphasis on very expensive preventive screening programmes for so-called primary prevention, is top heavy and is not cost effective. By health in India I mean the basic amenities for healthy living, viz., clean drinking water, food uncontaminated by animal and/or human excreta and a clean environment. These criteria collectively are referred to as primary health care for the purposes of this chapter.

By that definition, health care is very inexpensive compared to the enormous cost of treating diseases, the majority of which emanate from unhygienic surroundings and a lack of immunity in poorer sections. Poverty is the mother of all illnesses. One could see the dichotomy if one went into any five-star set-up. While it is heaven inside a hotel there, it is hell just outside that, but one has to have insight to see this. Mere eyesight, with or without glasses, would not help to see the squalor and the miserable state of those in hell.

Let us first concentrate on the health of our villagers which, if improved, could result in a quantum jump in our productivity and could, as a byproduct, reduce our birth rate as well, without any special effort. The usual plea of the powers-that-be is that doctors do not go to villages. We have to look into the root cause of doctors not going to or sticking to the villages. **Most of the present day doctors come from an urban background, even the small percentage of rural students get urbanized by the time they go through the arduous course in a medical school where the atmosphere is anything but rural. As such, the young medico is a stranger to a village and life therein**. He/she has no roots there. Neither is there any special incentive, although lip service is given to that on paper.

The singular reason why even a motivated and infracaninophilic young medico does not stick to the village has to do with his training. The latter is heavily loaded with technology. Clinical medicine, which flourished in the early part of this century, almost disappeared from the medical school environment after the sixties and seventies, when modern medicine went shopping to the market place riding piggyback on technology. If one picks up any textbook of medicine every disease starts with technology and ends with it. The medical student, therefore, gets convinced that technology is an integral part of diagnosis and treatment. We cannot fault him on that. Although there are studies even in the nineties that have elegantly shown that clinical medicine on the bedside is still the best, medi-business does not highlight it. "Do it" and "fix it" are the in-thing at medical schools. Many teachers are also convinced that without technology, medicine could never be practised.

The new medico in a village very soon gets frustrated and suffers from guilt as he thinks that he cannot deliver top class medical care. This guilt kills and they soon leave the village by hook or crook. It is not that they are any the less patriotic than our petty politicians who shout from house tops that if only doctors went to villages India would be heaven. In the bargain, if there were monetary allocations given to the village centre, politicians would find ways and means of siphoning their share of the booty! This hypocrisy kills even the last vestige of philanthropy in the rare breed of a passionate medico. Punishing them or making life difficult for them if they did not obey political orders is not the solution, as they cannot and would not practise medicine in a village, with a conscience, mainly because of their present day training. If the doctor wants a CAT scan for every headache and an ECHO for even muscular chest pain (that his boss at the school insisted upon), he would go mad soon in any village!

What do we need in the villages for health care that is both universal and primarily effective in a village population that has not been exposed to all the poisons that one gets in a large city atmosphere? **In addition to the trio of basic requirements like clean water, food and healthy surroundings, they need a good human being that could understand them in times of distress and empathize with them.** If that person could recognize rare instances of serious trouble, so that the sufferer may be taken without loss of precious time to the nearest hospital, most of the health care in the village could be looked after.

If this individual could also dole out harmless medicines for minor illness syndromes, which form the bulk of illnesses in the villages, our poor villagers would be ever happy and grateful. Family welfare, nutrition, and preventive vaccinations are other areas where this individual could make an impact. School health of the routine variety could also be added. This person would have to have a village background, and if possible, hail from the same village. He/she would be the friend, philosopher, and guide to our villagers winning their confidence, which in turn boosts their immune system!

Who could that person be? There is a move in the West now to empower nurses to become practitioners of medicine. These nurse practitioners have proven to be very useful in managing many of the common illness syndromes. These form the bulk of illnesses in society, anyway. A recent Canadian study showed that while a doctor sees one heart attack patient in the community he will have seen thirty thousand common illness syndromes.

India has many nursing schools and, if needed, they could be increased without much expenditure on infrastructure even in Taluka places with a hospital for hands-on training. It is possible to train our Auxiliary Nursing Midwives (ANMs) to double up as nurse practitioners in the villages. The scheme could be devised in such a way that girls with village background and some permanent interest in the village could be preferred.

We need not follow the set syllabus and teaching methods followed in the conventional schools. Interactive problem-based learning, with special emphasis on common illness syndromes, would be very useful. Their usual duties are taught side by side. Even the existing cadre could have a condensed course of a year to transform them into nurse practitioners. One need not worry about their misusing the drugs. They are given only very innocuous drugs, which even if given in larger than the usual doses or given to the wrong patient, should not produce serious problems. They could just handle analgesics, antipyretics, all the local topical creams, skin lotions, vitamins, innocuous sedatives, anti-asthma medications by the inhalation routes, and vaccines. Indian spices like ginger, onion, garlic, and pepper have been found to be very powerful anti-viral drugs for most common febrile conditions caused by viruses. They could not harm the patient, even when they are given to the wrong patient. The common cold research centre in London has advised people to eat Indian spicy food when they get a cold in the winter! We shy away from our own golden remedies.

I am sure these nurses would make better health keepers than highly trained doctor-technicians, the latter being doers and interventionists. They think it is below their dignity even to think of these minor illnesses. Many doctors have not heard of the minor illness syndromes. They are not being emphasized in the textbooks and are not being asked in their examinations. Today, conventional learning has become examination-oriented and not real-life-oriented. Once the examinations are over, what is learnt is conveniently forgotten until the next examination. Feverish cold, caused by a virus different from the one that causes common cold, is the cause of the largest sick-absenteeism in the world. I will be surprised to find a mention of that in any ordinary textbook of medicine for final MBBS students.

Do present day primary health centres serve their purpose? Let me give you the simple economics of these centers for the poor man in the village. The small town of Hiriradka, where I grew up, has a primary health centre covering many surrounding villages. My village is about five miles from the centre. When an elderly man has a headache in the village, he has to either walk that distance (or take a bus nowadays) to the town. His son becomes excited that his father is going to town and he accompanies him. The two go to the town in the morning. They wait for the doctor and their turn to be seen. Eventually, the old man might get an aspirin tablet for his tension headache, costing five paise. The old man and his son would have lost a day's work (one hundred fifty rupees), the bus fare comes to twenty rupees, and while in the town both of them eat in a restaurant (thirty rupees). In short, the aspirin tablet has cost the man two hundred rupees.

If the mountain of health care could go to Mohammed, things would be totally different. He could be given the aspirin by the nurse practitioner in the village itself. This is the way it should be in India where villages are far away from primary centers. In addition, the primary health centre of the existing variety could do very little compared to the capabilities of a qualified nurse. I am sure the powers-that-be would not like this idea as this takes away their ability to handle the large budget of the PHCs, from which they could siphon off their share of the booty. Unfortunately, we have become so corrupted that we have totally lost sight of the common good in the bargain.

I am told that in a particular area where the central government has allotted three hundred fifty crores to a particular cause, most of it is being siphoned off by the members of the committee, in addition to all the Babus from top to bottom. Nothing seems to have been spent for the real targets. Many of these people, I am told, think that it is not a bad idea to have a fake NGO in their relative's names to get the largesse from the allotment for their future safety. I am sure there would be opposition for the idea of a nurse practitioner scheme from all quarters. Some vested interests might argue that the nurse is not qualified to do what she is meant to do, little realizing that she is trained to perform adequately.

The government in India does not mind down-right quacks practising as registered medical practitioners. They should have to get a certificate from a revenue officer. This scheme would put an end to that kind of nefarious activity. Where we need strict vigilance we do not seem to have it. There are no rules to see that spurious drugs do not get sold as long as the manufacturer calls it Ayurveda. While we have too many rules for modern drugs, there are hardly any rules for "so-called" Ayurvedic drugs. The word Ayurveda is being misused for business by all and sundry. Genuine Ayurvedic preparations are so difficult to make that some manufacturers find it almost impossible these days, what with all the spurious ingredients in the market. We need to regulate drug manufacturing irrespective of the drug's label and do the same for the training requirements of RMPs.

A revenue officer certainly is not competent to certify a doctor as fit and be let loose on the gullible public. Most of these doctors might use harmful drugs, like steroids, for quick relief, without realizing the potential long-term dangers. This kind of activity goes on in our far-flung villages more than in cities. Good health care in the village would dampen an unfit doctor's enthusiasm to a great extent. Recent studies have shown how doctors going on strike in some countries has resulted in the death and disability rates going down remarkably! A five country study in Europe showed that in countries where there are more doctors per unit population, the health and longevity of the population was less than in those countries where there were fewer doctors for the same number of people. Higher doctor-patient ratio results in higher interventions and decreased health for the public. Doctors and hospitals have very little to do with a society's health!

I hope some thinking leaders in society would give serious thought to this idea. Let there be a national debate and something fruitful might emerge. I do not want to claim that this is a perfect idea. We could always modify and see how it fits. While the affluent West wants to change from their top-heavy medical system to something less expensive, we in India do not bother to audit our systems at all. Once put in place they are presumed to be good for all times to come and under all circumstances. "Let noble thoughts come to us from all sides," says the Rig Veda.

> **I don't give them hell. I just tell the truth and they think it is hell.**
>
> *—Harry S Truman*

Further Reading

- Hegde BM. *Ancient Wisdom in Science and Health.* Delhi College of Physicians and Surgeons, New Delhi. 2003.

CHAPTER 17

The Patient that Changed my Life

I do not know a better training for a writer than to spend some years in the medical profession-the doctor, especially hospital doctor, sees (human nature) bare.

—Somerset Maugham in *The Summing Up*

One learns everyday in life, as life itself is the best school. "No one can teach anyone anything that he/she does not already know" wrote Alexis Carroll. I strongly feel that each one of us learns for himself/herself, if only one keeps all senses alert all the time. One incident that supports this feeling, accidentally changed my life. It was the beginning of my real education. My schooling had come in the way of my education even though, in the beginning, I did not go to school at the elementary level. I did learn a lot at home from my own mother and my surroundings. I was quite at home in that environment in my native village. After I started going to school my education came to a standstill. I became a robot, trying to learn all that the books and the teachers' notes had to teach me!

I started life in Mangalore city as a consultant and a junior teacher in the year 1964. Young as I was, I was very confident of everything. There is an old saying that "the young know everything, middle age suspects everything; but old age believes everything." Now I can certify that the statement is one hundred per cent true. To cap it, I must also have been a bit arrogant because I was considered a very good student in the conventional sense of the term. I had the best of training in cardiology in some of the best places in the world—The Middlesex and National Heart Hospitals, London, and the Peter Brent Brigham Hospital of the Harvard Medical School.

The incident I mean to speak of involved a man named Devanna (not his real name) who was a young man in his mid 30s, seemingly quite healthy and fit. He was having his regular check ups and went through all the routine rigmarole that we doctors advise patients to go through. He was brought to our hospital in the early hours of a November morning almost dead after having suffered a massive heart attack. I was called in but could do precious little to save him. His young wife was in deep shock, naturally. She could not accept this lightning blow to her married life. In that dazed state she was rolling on the floor in the ICU, holding my ankle tightly asking me the most difficult question in my life: "Why did my husband die, doctor?" I could have given her a long lecture on "how" her husband died, but had no answer for her question "why".

Strange it was, but I, for the first time, felt that I was totally incompetent as I could not answer a simple question from the bereaved wife. That set me thinking and a realization dawned on me that I was ignorant about most of the things that happened around me. It was a rude awakening. Little did I realize that all those encomiums that I earned in college and school were mere decorations for collecting information about the human body and its function, but the real working of this universe and of the human body in the universe were still enigmas to me.

I had my first lesson in true education-humility. I was reminded of TS Eliot's poem:

"Where is the wisdom we seem to have lost in Knowledge?
And where is the knowledge, we seem to have lost in information?"

Knowledge dwells in heads replete with thoughts of other men while wisdom dwells in heads attentive to their own. I went in search of my own head and continue to do so today. I searched religions, philosophy, theology, our scriptures, quantum physics, and even teleology deeply. That is where I found some solace and some vague answers to the question "why". I happened to read an excellent novel based on a true story that occurred in 1844 in Peru. It was the famous American author Thornton Wilder's *The Bridge on San Luis Rey*, written in 1927. The story revolves round the unexpected collapse of the famous bridge across the huge gorge dividing Lima, the capital of Peru, from the mainland, which everyone in Peru had to cross at sometime or another.

The bridge was built by the Incas and was supposed to never break. Yet, break it did one afternoon in 1844, killing five people, one of whom was a small innocent child. The grieving mother of the child is consoled by a wise old lady of the neighborhood. Wilder makes some very pertinent points in that dialogue about the existence of two worlds—the world of the dead and the world of the living—both connected by an unbreakable bridge of *human love*. If one were to love those near and dear after they pass away as long as one still lives, death loses its importance. It was a great philosophic thought and gave me solace.

Similarly, Buddhism gives the best solution to the problem. Gautama Buddha, the enlightened one, thought that death is not the end at all; it is just the change from one state to another. Where, then is the problem in death? Death is not the end but a part, an essential part, of life itself. The subatomic world connects all of us together and binds us with this universe: death loses its horror in that background. Quantum physics is very close to the *Sanaathana Dharma*—the ageless wisdom of India's hoary past—in this way.

It was at this stage that I chanced upon that precious paper by Charles Sherrington, the famous physiologist, who had discovered many new facets of human physiology. Sherrington was just 42 years old when he was appointed Professor of Physiology at the Liverpool University in 1899. In his inaugural address he had this to say: "Positive sciences would not answer the question "why"; they could, at best, answer "how" or "how much", but not "why" A physiologist could answer as to how does the heart contract but will never be able to say why does the heart contract." How true, indeed.

Medical science, along with all other natural sciences, lost its very moorings in 1742, when a young boy aged 17, believed to be a great mathematician, Rene Descartes, proclaimed to the world *cogito ergo sum*. He, for the first time, cut off the human mind from the human body, calling them by different names—*res cogitans* and *res extensa*. Retrospectively, this was the greatest tragedy of modern reductionist science. The dynamic universe never follows reductionist linear laws but goes by holistic principles. The human mind is not only an integral part of the human body. It is the very core of every cell in the human body at the sub-atomic quantum level. All diseases and all our problems start in the mind. The symptoms are felt in the body (soma) since the mind cannot be seen or imagined by patients. Reductionism and deterministic predictabilities are only myths in this universe.

I have been looking at medical science more critically since the day Devanna passed away and have been able to discover the hypocrisy of most of what we preach or do to our hapless victims—the patients. I have also been trying my best to expose these hidden dangers of modern medicine with the view to helping young doctors separate the wheat from the chaff. In the last fifty years, medicine has been hijacked by technology and taken from the bedside to the market place. The latter has made modern medicine only a dream for the majority of the people in this world. It is prohibitively expensive and top heavy. The dangers of this kind of inhuman medicine have to be dinned into the heads of new entrants to the profession before they get converted by the prevailing situation. Prince Charles, the heir to the British throne, had recently summed up the present scenario in his own inimitable style thus: "Modern medicine, for all its breathtaking achievements, is slightly off balance like the Tower of Pisa." He couldn't have been more accurate. Although I had quoted Price Charles before, I have done it again to impress upon the young medicos that might read this book. I always quote great people to reinforce my ideas. Great people are heard and seen!

I must admit that I have now realized that the greatest discovery of this century is the discovery of man's ignorance. At least, as far as I am concerned, this is absolutely true. *Learning is a life long process and there is no end to it.* Life teaches man all that he needs to know, but man has to be awake all the time to learn. We have all come from that great source of energy—the creator—from whom we can draw all the energy that we need to push ahead in life. If we have the **intention and will**, we can all achieve great things in life. The power of intention is enormous. One has to be a student all his/her life.

> I like to see doctors cough,
> What kind of human being
> Would grab all your money
> Just when you're down?
> I'm not saying they enjoy this:
> "Sorry, Mr. Rodriguez, that's it,
> No hope! You might as well
> hand over your wallet." Hell no,
> they'd rather be playing golf
> and swapping jokes about our feet.
>
> —James Tate, Contemporary American poet,
> on doctors, in his book *Viper Jazz*

FURTHER READING

- Denise Gellene, Tenet Says Its Redding Hospital May Be Barred From Medicare, *Los Angeles Times* 5th Sep. 2003.
- Hegde BM. The science of medicine. *J Assosc Physci India* 1998; 46: 896-97.
- Pickering WG. Does medical treatment mean patient benefit? *Lancet* 1996;347: 379–80.

CHAPTER 18

Medical Consultation

It is a secret known but to few, yet no small use in the conduct of life, that when you fall into a man's conversation, the first thing you should consider is whether he has a greater inclination to hear you or that you should hear him.

—*Steele*

The crux of medical consultation—a patient meeting a doctor—is where a **human being** who is ill or imagines being ill, meets another **human being** in whom the ill person has confidence. This coming together of two human beings with mutual confidence is the apex of all else in the field of medical care delivery. The technology, medical school, laboratory, therapy, and surgery flow from this summit. The patient-doctor relationship and the resultant trust in each other is the main stimulus for the body's immune system, which eventually heals all ills. Medical interventions with drugs and surgery are only the means to this end where the repair mechanism is set in motion to heal the sickness. Drugs and surgery are needed to remove any gross impediments in the process of healing, but the healing depends solely on the repair mechanism of the body, which in turn, depends on the **faith** that the patient has in his/her doctor.

Modern hi-tech sub-specialized medicine lacks this very basis of healing. Consequently, in those developed countries where technology and specialization have reached dizzying heights with the patient becoming just another case for intervention, doctors are becoming dangerous to patients. Any human being who sees a doctor becomes a patient from then on, rarely to become a human being again, thanks to our definition of normal ity which includes many normal humans in the category of patients, the so-called false positives. We do not let the "well" alone. Three studies strongly bring out these facts.

The recent *Institute of Medicine* report in the US ranks doctors and hospitals as the **third** most important cause of death there, with only heart attacks and cancers preceding doctors in that order of importance. The fourth cause of death in the US seems to be the side effects (ADR) of known drugs prescribed by doctors. The US is the last but one in the ranking for good medical care among the 14 developed countries surveyed recently. Japan, where the doctor-patient ratio is the lowest among the 14 developed countries, ranks the best. The report cites the lack of good family doctors in the US as the cause of this sad state of affairs. The last study, and the last straw on the camel's back, is the report from Israel. Doctors there went on strike a couple of years ago for three months demanding higher pay. An audit now shows that death rates sharply plummeted during the strike, only to come back to the normal levels when doctors came back to work. Morticians, whose business went down significantly during the strike, had brokered peace between the striking doctors and the government in Israel!

Doctors, who have to be the placebo (Latin=I please) effect in the healing process have instead become nocebo (dangerous) doctors. The developing countries have a lesson to learn from all these studies. We must build a very strong base of well-trained family physicians that should form the strong foundation of medical care delivery. Hi-tech specialists should only be called in to intervene after a decision about intervention has been taken by the family doctor, based purely on the patient's need, at the end of the consultation. The specialist should never be in direct first contact with the patients. There is the danger of intervention rates going up unnecessarily, replicating the experience of the developed countries.

Many doctors and most lay people have a misconception that hi-tech investigations are needed for arriving at a good diagnosis. The truth, however, is otherwise. A recent prospective, double blind, and computerized study in London showed that **eighty per cent of the accurate final diagnoses and one hundred per cent of the future management strategies could be arrived at, at the end of listening to the patient and reading the old records, if at all. This is refined only 4% more by elaborate examinations and only 8% more by all investigations, including the positron emission tomography!** We are back to square one. It was a great medical brain of the last century, Lord Platt, who wrote in 1949: "If you listen to your patient long enough he/she would tell you what is wrong with him/her." This has been proven true by the London study mentioned above. Interestingly, the study was conducted by five of Lord Platt's old students at the University College Hospital London, who now are the main pillars of medical education in the UK in different medical schools.

In this scenario, it is our duty to educate the public (potential patients) about their responsibility in this coming together of two human beings with mutual confidence, the medical consultation. If the patient does not share the responsibility, the outcome may not be the same. The time of paternalism in medicine, where the doctor was considered omnipotent, has to be replaced by partnership in medicine, where the final outcome of any illness depends both on the doctor and the patient. The public must also be taught that doctors are not infallible and that they could also make mistakes. In that setting the patient realizes the possibility of mistakes and if the doctor is honest about any mishaps the chances of legal problems could also be sorted out amicably. Again, it is the mutual trust that should be the basis of this partnership. Like any other partnership, in order to last long, both parties must believe in giving and not getting alone. Money should not be the sole motivator for the doctor. Gratitude of a patient cured, comforted, or consoled should be the greatest reward. Money will automatically come when the patient is satisfied—the less fortunate being more honest than the rich and the powerful!

What should the patient do when he/she meets with his/her family doctor? He/she should tell the doctor all that he/she knows about the symptoms, the environment of his/her living and working, anxieties, worries and fears, family matters, as well as the work environment: peers, superiors, and inferiors at work. Medical effort is all about allaying the patient's anxiety of death and disability and the doctor's anxiety of having done enough or not. **One should not forget to tell the doctor about any drug that one is taking, even if they are food supplements, vitamins, herbal drugs, homeopathic, or any other "insignificant" drug.** Please remember that a good 25% of the hospital admissions are due to adverse drug reactions, unbeknownst to patients and doctors. The public should be urged to never keep anything from their family doctor when they are not well. "Good" habits like smoking and alcohol intake should also be told in detail to the doctor. One's fears, obsessions, worries, and feelings about others and even their dreams might provide a clue to the diagnosis. One should never ever think that the doctor is a God and would be able to fish out the diagnosis with his/her training at the medical school. The final diagnosis depends more on the patient than on the doctor. An intelligent patient is an asset to a good doctor.

Many would think that the illiterate poor people will not be able to assist their doctors in this scenario. Far from truth! Many, if not all, of these "so-called" illiterate but well educated people, with their innate wisdom and intuition, will be able to give out more details to their doctors in the villages where a diagnosis is a better possibility in the majority of patients. Our only problem in the villages is the inability of young doctors to work there, not so much because of the lack of facilities for them to live there but because the present day westernized hi-tech based medical education does not equip them well for being let loose on the gullible people in the village. Students learn more by their teacher's example on the bed side rather than the teachers' pontifications in the class-rooms. Today's teachers do not take time to talk to, leave alone listen to, the patients, and they base their diagnosis only on technology. So their students would want the same in the village where it is not available. A conscientious young doctor feels guilty in such a set-up that he might miss the diagnosis because of the lack of scopes and scanners! This has to change by innovative tailoring of the present teaching-learning process in the medical schools. This is the long and the short of good doctoring.

He who sedulously attends, pointedly asks, calmly speaks, coolly answers, and ceases when he has no more to say, is in the possession of some of the best requisites of man.
—Lavater

FURTHER READING

- Michel Foucault. *The Birth of the Clinic.* 1972 Vintage Publications.
- Linden W, Stossel C and Maurice J. Psycho-social interventions for patients with CAD. *Arch Intern Med.* 1996; 156: 745–752.
- Department of Health (2004 November) *Choosing health: Making healthier choices easier.* CM 6374 London: The Stationary Office. 207 p.
- Eisenberg L (1984) Rudolf Ludwig Karl Virchow, where are you, snow that we need you? *Am J Med* 77: 524–532.
- Starfield B. Is US medicine the best in the world? *JAMA* 2000; 284: 483–488

CHAPTER 19

Medical Teleology

Positive sciences do not answer the question, "why?" They could, at best, answer "how" or "how much". One could explain how a patient died, in great detail. We enjoy the famous CPC's so much that we lose sight of the fact that under similar circumstances another human being might not have died! One young man at thirty five could drop down dead instantaneously of a massive myocardial infarction, while another seventy year old man/woman could have similar infarct and go on to recover and live a full life! Why did the first one die? When people survive doctors claim credit. Medical business also would want to believe that medical interventions keep people alive. On the contrary, a recent strike by doctors in Israel, where they refused to interfere except in dire emergencies, mortality and morbidity came down significantly. Even in emergencies, the scenario was not very much different. The war casualties of Vietnam and Falklands were audited in a recent study. Whereas Vietnam had the best of emergency facilities with helicopters and a hi-tech base hospital in Saigon, the wounded soldiers in Falklands were left to the vagaries of the cold snow for want of facilities for even up to 6–12 hours without intervention. However, the per capita mortality was decidedly in favor of Falklands!

I have been in this business for nearly half a century, studying human health and disease from the first day of my joining the Stanley Medical College in Madras in 1956 and am still a student of human health and ill health. What amazes me is the lack of *thinking* researchers in the field. Most of us seem to go with the flow. All most all of us are swept off our feet by the hi-tech hurricane originating on either side of the Atlantic Ocean. We are made to believe that there is "ne plus ultra"—no more beyond—the hi-tech world. It also makes good business sense! Medical establishment, which originated as an altruistic noble calling, has now turned into the biggest money spinner industry, attracting the big multinational sharks to get into five star hospitals business. "Never make money in the sick room," wrote Hippocrates, the founding father of modern medicine. Medical establishment probably is the biggest single headache free industrial enterprise these days. Egged on by moneylenders, it also helps the unscrupulous to launder their black money in this business. There is no harm if all this is done to help people. To cap it, we have the new class of man eating sharks who live on sale of human organs.

There is another face to all these claptrap. People who get involved in this business, the doers, get lot of publicity and patronage by the powers-that-be. On the sidelines are the greater and richer players in the drama. They are the technology manufacturers and the drug barons. They have been shown to even invent new diseases lately to sell their wares, aided and abetted by the greedy 'doctors'. One of the most recent new diseases is the *female impotence* invented to sell sildenafil (Viagra). Male population being less than the female and most elderly males having contraindications for Viagra, the company that made a net profit of $11.2 billion last year thinks that if females, especially those who are young, were induced to take it the profit might be ten times more! Epidemiologists are another class who cause epidemics by frightening healthy people and making them fall into the drug company nets. We have a lot of them predicting the unpredictable epidemics of diabetes, high blood pressure, and vascular diseases, while the truth is that there has not been even one per cent **absolute increase** in the incidence of vascular diseases in the last one century! Larger populations, people living to middle ages and beyond because of the decrease in killer infections in childhood, increased disease awareness, the diagnostic wrong labeling of the apparently healthy, and the ageing population that naturally qualifies for degenerative diseases cause the apparent increase. Fear in the minds of the public increases their sugar level, fat level, as also their blood pressures. Thus they fall into the "doctor-thinks-you-have-a-disease" label basket. This kind of routine screening of apparently healthy people has been shown to be dangerous! Who cares as long as it makes our tills move?

Divine interventionalists, another menace to healthy people in society, claim that they intervene early to prevent a future catastrophe. The truth, though, is different. No one could predict the future of a dynamic human system. Audits have shown most of these interventions in very poor light. The big seller, coronary bypass surgery, as also its close cousin angioplasty, have benefited only a small percentage of recipients, especially those with intractable symptoms. Even early surgery for certain cancers has been shown not to have helped the poor victims! Some of these interventions have attracted more dangerous and even fatal complications. Early bypass surgery immediately after a heart attack has been shown to have increased four fold the stroke incidence in those patients within the next six months, and most of these strokes had been fatal!

The expensive drugs for chronic "doctor-thinks-you-have diseases", like high blood pressure, asymptomatic hyperglycemia and blood vessel and joint diseases have all increased total mortality when followed up beyond five years! Hormone replacement therapy (HRT) after menopause, oral calcium to prevent osteoporosis, and long term use of vitamins instead of natural sources of these vital amines, fruits and vegetables, have all come to grief on long-term audits!

That said, let us try and understand human health and healthy existence on this planet using the existing knowledge in the field of science. Medical science, like many other conventional reductionist sciences, is a game of uncertainties. Newer quantum mechanics has shown that the sub-atomic particles do what they do only when we look at them. When we are not looking at them only God knows what they do. Despite knowing the half-life of the decaying atom in Erwin Schrödinger's cat hypothesis experiment, the reality of the cat being alive or dead inside the closed box, depended ultimately on the observer looking into the box to find out. The chance of the cat dying as per the predictions was only fifty-fifty. We are now back one full circle to the beginning of the doctrine of probabilities of Blaise Pascal. So everything in the realm of science is in the eye of the beholder. If one changes the tinted statistical scientific glasses in the field of human illness and wellness, one would quickly realize our fallacies. It is not a wonder that in one year, three hundred thousand people died in the US due to medical mistakes alone. A good quarter of the hospital admissions there were due to iatrogenic diseases!

Teleologically, man is built to last. Nature has provided enough in-built safely measures and even repair mechanisms to keep the organism going on for a full life span. Of course, ageing would catch up as time passes and death, the only certainty, genetically programmed into each one of us, is the final outcome. The only risk factor for death is life. Nature does not intend that we become immortal. If people do not die where is the place on this planet for all of us? Even the exaggerated claims of egoistic scientists claiming to clone man have received a big blow when a sobered down Ian Wilmot had to euthanase 'Dolly" his first creation to send her to meet Wilmot's maker!

Man never had any illnesses in the sustenance economies of yore. This was shown in a scientific study of the Iannus in an island off the coast of Saskachiwan in Canada. Monetary economy with its greed, hatred, jealousy and, the killer competitive ethos, changed all that. To cap it we have changed the symbiotic relationships between all the creatures in Nature and have spoiled, in addition, the environment to make it more conducive to create human illnesses. Recent studies have shown that even small amounts (declared safe by scientists) of background radiation could be dangerous to human health. Despite all that our built-in repair systems, the autonomic nervous system and the immune shield, help us to overcome diseases most of the time. Only when they fail, man suffers pain and other symptoms of disease. If one studies the microscopic world of heart muscle cells after an infarct one wonders at the marvel of nature in trying to remodel the ventricle. Rarely when this process fails, we doctors could help and hope to get temporary reprieve for the victim. Earlier interventions, using drugs that block either of the above protective systems, have been shown to be dangerous. This is also true after grave injury as shown in the Falklands war study.

In conclusion, the existing wisdom (not knowledge) in science in general and medical science in particular would convince any thinking student of human health that doctors, drugs and technology should only be used to assist Nature when it fails (that is when patient manifests symptoms) to cure rarely, comfort mostly, but to console always. Doctors should stop playing God. Doctors should not deceive themselves by the industrial claptrap to think that every human ill has a pill and they have the power to intervene in healthy people to keep them here for ever. Only a philosophic teleological outlook in the medical field would be a boon to mankind. Before you want my blood for writing this, stop and think. Even intercessory prayer has been shown in elegant experiments to help heart attack patients! If one treats Nature as our mother she would nourish us, if abused she would kick us.

Further Reading

- Siegel-Itzkovich J. Doctors' strike in Israel may be good health. *BMJ* 2000; 320:1561.
- Moynihan R, Heath I, Henry D. Selling Sickness: the pharmaceutical industry and disease mongering. *BMJ* 2002; 324: 886–891.
- Stehabens W.
- Stewart Brown S and Farmer A. Screening could seriously damage your health. *BMJ* 1997; 314: 533–534

- Hux JE and Naylor CD. In the eye of the beholder. *Arch Intern Med.* 1995; 155: 2277–2280.
- Josefson D. Early bypass surgery increases the risk of stroke. *BMJ* 2001; 323: 185.
- Beral V, Banks E, Reeves G. Evidence from randomised trials on the long term effects of hormone replacement therapy. *Lancet* 2002; 360: 942–944.
- Gribbin J. *In Search of the Schrödinger's cat.* 1984. Black Swan Publishers, London.
- Hegde BM. God Forgotten- Man Sleighted. *Lancet* (accepted, yet to be published)

CHAPTER 20

Limits of Science

Science becomes dangerous only when it imagines that it has reached its goal.

—George Bernard Shaw (1856–1950)
in *Doctor's Dilemma*

Scientists make the tall claim that science and scientific outlook have taken mankind forward in the last one hundred odd years. What provoked me to write this piece is that little wonderful book, *Limits of Science,* by the great scientist and Nobel laureate, Sir Peter Medawar. Anyone who questions the above rhetoric is dubbed as superstitious or downright illogical, in addition to being unscientific. Rational thinking is said to be the key to good living and wisdom. How I wish it were that simple! Rationality, per force, has to have its limitations. Rational thinking is based on the inputs from five senses and possibly some degree of "knowledge" derived from one's past experience. All these do not come in lumpsums but in bits and pieces. Pascal was the first to proclaim that there are two important aspects of man's life that are vital to his actions. **First is to exclude reason in his dealings; and the second is to believe that there is nothing beyond reason.** Going back hundreds of years, this thinker could have foreseen the truth of his statement despite the fact that the present scientific advances that we swear by did not exist then. He is not far off the mark even today.

Rational thinking and scientific outlook have enormous limitations. When you look beyond reason you get an insight into Nature's functioning better. **Nature has its reasons always, but our reason cannot explore them many a time.** How else can one feel love, hatred, jealousy etc., in life?

None of them can be measured in scientific terms. One could experience love but not be able to see love and measure its dimensions. To deny the effects of intense feeling of love for one's beloved or oneself is to deny the truth. If "science is measurement and measurement is science" as defined by Marie Curie, love as an emotion does not exist at all. No one has seen the wind, but when the trees dance and bend the wind is passing by, wrote Christina, the American poetess.

Similarly, there are a lot of things that one can only feel but cannot see and measure. The problem with mankind today is intolerance for other's views. Rousseau was despised by many of his peers for his strong and unconventional views. His life was in danger. Voltaire came to his rescue and asked Rousseau to stay with him to avoid any harm. Eventually when Rousseau did come, Voltaire told him, "I do not agree with a single word of what you say, but I shall defend to my last breath your right to say what you want to say."

That is the kind of tolerance that would take mankind forward. Science, if anything, has taken mankind backwards, if one critically looks at it philosophically, and has pushed him to the brink of self-destruction. Is not the threat of nuclear war from terrorists based on scientific data? Is not the anthrax fear in the USA born out of complicated scientific research to get resistant germs to fight wars? Is not the ever-present threat of chemical warfare based on science?

Recently, when doctors went on strike in Israel the death rate and morbidity fell significantly there, only to bounce back to the original levels when there was peace between the striking doctors and the government. It is to be noted that morticians, whose business all but disappeared when the strike was on, brokered peace between the striking doctors and the government! The so-called evidence-based medicine, when looked at carefully, is only evidence burdened and makes life that much more difficult for both the doctor and the patient. This is because scientific evidence gathered need not have a linear relationship to what happens inside the human body. The latter is run by the human mind, which is scientifically unfathomable. There are so many imponderables in Nature that one cannot answer all the questions in Nature with the help of science alone. There are many things outside the realm of science, which are beyond the explanatory capacity of science.

Any intolerance is the beginning of terrorism and "scientific intolerance" is one such. Scientific terrorism could be more lethal than the present day political terrorism. If allowed to go beyond control it could destroy mankind forever. Let us look at some happenings that science will never be able to gauge. Years ago Leonard Leibovici showed that "remote, retroactive, intercessory prayer could do wonders for patient recovery in hospitals." A positivist that he was, he went a step further to urge doctors to include prayer in their armamentarium. He also gave evidence to show how scurvy could be controlled hundreds of years before the discovery of vitamin C, as shown by James Lind.

The prayer theme was taken to great scientific heights by a recent study in an American University hospital in a well controlled, randomized, triple-blind (the patient, his treating doctor and the relatives are kept in the dark) prospective study of heart attack patients. The prayed for group had very significant fall in all parameters of the illness in a coronary care set up. This was replicated in patients who had severe infective fevers in another milestone study. Konotey-Ahulu documented some unexplainable deaths in his hospital in Africa (very thoroughly studied even after postmortem) where medical science could not give any explanation. Recitation of the Rosary, which derives its origin from the Tibetan monks, brought to the West via Arabs and other crusaders, and the yoga mantras that are well known in India, have been elegantly shown to reduce the rate of breathing, which results in significant improvement in the patients' illness. Yogic breathing is shown to lower elevated blood pressure, and many other cardiac parameters like aortic pressure, pulmonary artery pressure, the ventricular ejection fraction etc., in those with severe heart failure. It bestows the immeasurable added benefit of "tranquility of mind".

Studies in America showed that Chinese and Japanese Americans had significantly higher death rates on the 4th of every month. This was not seen in the White races. The Chinese and the Japanese believe the 4th to be very inauspicious day of the month. Another milestone study in London showed that Friday the 13th was definitely dangerous for at least fifty per cent of Britons who dared to go out and work that day. The other fifty per cent stayed home on those days: the really superstitious. The conclusion of the study was that Friday the 13th is definitely bad for at least one half of the British population.

If one is a conscientious medical scientist and observes patients very closely one will discover many such inexplicable feats happening almost every day in a busy clinical setting. I call them "butterfly effects", the phrase having been borrowed from Edward Lorenz of weather predictions fame. It was only after Lorenz got all the bouquets for his discovery of the method of predicting the weather that he discovered, to his surprise, that accurate prediction of the weather is impossible. He then propounded the butterfly effect. If one wants to know the limitations of science one should study human beings in distress, where the butterfly effect is the rule rather than an exception. Of course, doctors have been predicting the unpredictable all along.

One unforgettable incident comes to mind. One of my patients, whom I had known in my professional capacity for a very long time, was the priest of a very famous temple in Malanad area of Karnataka State in India. He was an authentic scholar of ancient Indian wisdom and was venerated by his people. He managed his temple affairs with total dedication. His temple was an example for others. When this incident occurred he was well past ninety years of age but was very alert mentally as well as physically. His wife, who was in her 80s, was admitted under my care for a heart attack (inferior infarct, a milder variety with good outcome). When she was progressively improving, on the third day he made a strange request to me. He wanted her to be discharged that very day, as he was sure that she would meet her maker the following day at 12 noon or so. I was non-plussed but, knowing him as I did to be very authentic, I was in a "scientific" dilemma. Ultimately he took her against medical advice. His argument was that she should not die in a hospital.

I was shocked to learn from their son that the patient was in good shape at 11.55 am and she drank some water and died without any distress at 12 noon. I could not bring myself to believe this whole episode until after a year, when the old man wanted to see me to thank me. He told me that he was going to die on a particular day at a given time and wanted all his children and grandchildren around him at that time. This prediction made me curious. He did keep his word and the end came as he had predicted. He had all his people around and slept on a banana leaf on the floor minutes before breathing his last! I have no scientific explanation even now. He was a great astrologer himself and had done very deep study of all the great works in that area. He had a reputation of being an authentic astrologer, in addition to his philanthropy – all for free!

This single episode is only one example of the many paranormal phenomena that one observes in day-to-day medical practice. Konotey Ahulu's episodes are stranger than mine are, though. Maybe they are culturally different; he was practising in Africa. I know what *Erik the Genius* would say. Since he is an intellectual and a know-all scientist, he would label all our experiences as anecdotal. Of course, they are anecdotal, but it is anecdotes that make us wiser and not arrogant. Any knotty problem, when looked at more carefully, becomes more complicated. Great minds of yore knew this very well. Albert Einstein, during his last days, wrote: "I do not believe that this world is a wonder; I think it is a wonderful wonder." Stephen Hawkins wrote: "I do not believe that there is God; if there is one I do not want him to interfere with my work."

What Doctors Don't Get to Study in Medical School

Wisdom is not just the sum total of the inputs from our five senses. There is more to it than what meets the eye. The effects of prayer on illness, the placebo-doctor effect on the human immune system, the "will to live" feeling that keeps people going despite intolerable pain and disability, and many other such scientifically proven methods of giving relief to the suffering make one believe in the possibilities beyond hypothesis refutation and measurements.

Science, like any other human activity, should have its limitations. It would be foolhardy to believe that science is the be-all and end-all of human wisdom. Very far from it. What we know is probably a very small fraction of what there is to know. This is the best education scientifically given in school: Live and let live. While one could have one's views, one should be tolerant of others views as well and be ready to examine them without any prejudices. That would be progress and that alone can rid this world of all kinds of terrorism. One who understands science very well alone realizes the depth of his ignorance. **The genuine rationalist is one who has understood the limitations of reason.** Positive sciences, at best, could answer questions like "how" or "how much." Positive sciences will never be able to answer the question "why". The answer to the question "why" needs the knowledge of **the limits of science.**

> *Qua deus hanc mundi temperet arte domum,*
> *Qua venit exoriens, qua deficit, unde coactis*
> *Cornibus in plenum menstrua luna redit,*
> *Unde salo superant venti, quid flamine captet*
> *Eurus, et in nubes unde perennis aqua?*

—Michael de Montaigne in The Essays

("By what artifice God governs this world, our home; where the moon comes from, where she does go and how she does bring her horns together month after month and so grow full; whence the gales spring which rule the salty sea, and what dominion does the South Wind enjoy; whence come those waters which are ever in the clouds?"—translation by MA Screech)

Further Reading

- Peter Medawar. *Limits to Science.*
- Steven Milloy. *Science without Sense.* Cato Institute, Washington DC. 1993.
- Michel de Montaigne. *The Essays* (English translation by Prof. Screech).

CHAPTER 21

Modern Medicine and Quantum Physics

Anyone who is not shocked by quantum theory has not understood it.

—*Niels Bohr (1885–1962)*

Biology, in general, is still in search of its Holy Grail, leave alone drinking from it! Medicine is still to go a long way. Unfortunately, most of us, both within and outside the system, believe that we have a strong scientific foundation for our craft. When the controlled studies were first invented, knowledgeable people in the medical field thought that the last word in the history of medicine's progress had been written. There is nothing more to worry about, they thought. In reality, we have an evidence-burdened system in place of what is popularly known as evidence-based medicine. We go around bashing every other system of medicine as unscientific. For a change, let us try and understand the science behind modern medicine, if there is any.

What is the reality? There is no reality at all. What we have believed is only a mirage. When we compare two cohorts of age and sex matched human beings, we are only able to match their phenotypes, that too a microscopic part of the whole phenotype, *while time evolution in a human system depends on the total initial knowledge of the human being*. The genotype and the all-pervading consciousness, are beyond the reach of present day assessment. We presume that our randomization takes care of all the missing links. There is very little similarity between two individuals; even binovular twins are not identical. When the two groups are not identical, the end result of our controlled studies will, per force, go wrong. We have been drawing wrong conclusions all along and have been predicting the future of individuals based on this faulty foundation. In short, we have been predicting the unpredictable. That is the main reason why every single long-term cohort comparison has thrown up surprise findings.

That apart, the human body does not work in bits and pieces. It works as a whole and in tune with the environment. Our reductionist science of studying the cell or intracellular structures and then projecting the information on to the organ and the whole body will have to go wrong, anyway! Recent studies of human physiology have brought out three rhythms in the human body—the circadian, ultradian and the infradian. The last one has a longer than 24-hours cycle. The one prominent rhythm that falls in this category is the menstrual cycle. The menstrual cycle is ultimately under the control of the gravitational effect of the Moon on the cortical cells that stimulate the pituitary. The latter, in turn, sends impulses to the other endocrine glands! Simple hormone replacement therapy could, therefore, not be harmless, as shown by more recent studies.

Whenever we are stuck with our controlled studies, many leaders take shelter under the umbrella of statistics. Basically, statistics are used in medical research to rule out the possibility of chance playing a role in the final outcome. That is the limited role of statistics in medical research. At the same time, statistics could be used as the whipping boy to get out of any inconvenient research situation that might not fit in with our hypothesis, especially in drug studies. "Intention-to-treat-analysis" is one such catch that could be used to confuse the novitiates. The underlying problem is the large amount of money being sunk by drug lords in isolating the powerful molecule in the laboratory to begin with. When found to be useful in animals they go for human studies hoping to get similar results. If the results are not to their liking, instead of writing off that huge sum, they get enough people to explain the variance with difficult statistical jargon to confuse the medical team. The latter are mostly ignorant of the nuances of intricate statistical jugglery. This applies to many of the heroic surgical feats as well. Prominent among them are cardiac interventions and cancer "cure" methods. Some of these procedures are big money spinners. In short, the present day medical science seems to be guided mainly by monetary considerations rather than altruism.

The Real Science

Medicine was accepted as a science in the 12th century Europe and was clubbed with physics, chemistry and biology. Our research since then has been based on those three disciplines. However, in the early part of the twentieth century, physics realized that the laws of "*deterministic predictability*" did not work in reality. In truth, there was no reality in this Universe. A classic example is the Nobel Prize given to JJ Thomson in the year 1907 for showing that electrons were particles. Thirty years later his own son JG Thomson received his Nobel in 1937 for showing that electrons were waves. Both were right and both were wrong! They both came from the world famous Cavendish Laboratory of the Cambridge University. Most of the physics Nobel prizes those days went to those working at Cavendish.

This was the birth of the new quantum physics. Some of the great names to remember are those of Werner Heisenberg, Erwin Schrödinger, Max Planck, Niels Bohr, Paul Dirac and Born, although both Isaac Newton and Albert Einstein had contributed to the development of the new thinking indirectly. Albert Einstein, though, could not stomach the new thinking in the field till he died. He dubbed Schrödinger's hypothesis as "some sort of a mathematical trick."

The tragedy was that medicine did not fork off to follow the less traveled route in physics. Rather, it continued to follow the laws of *deterministic predictability*. The human body does not follow the latter rules.

$$2 \times 3 <NOT> 3 \times 2$$
(inside the human system)
because
$$p \times q <NOT> q \times p$$
(Heisenberg's uncertainty equation)

In any given situation these calculations are not really true, but in ordinary situations in the macro world, we do not realize the errors because the margin of error is very, very small as Δp and Δq are usually much larger than the Planck's constant **h ÷ 2Π**, roughly of the order of **10** $^{-27}$ (Δ is the symbol mathematicians use for minor errors).

But at the quantum level, and even in the human body, these minor errors might be very serious. Even an error of one in a million might result in catastrophic end results as time evolves. The other name for this game is the "butterfly effect" of Edward Lorenz. After having been crowned as the inventor of weather prediction methods, Lorenz, a physics professor at Berkley University, was sorry that the small details of weather predictions of the immediate future, as also the finer aspects of the predictions, rarely come correct. He exclaimed that even if a butterfly were to move its wings in Beijing in China, the air disturbance could develop into a storm in New York after a month!

The dynamic human body, driven continuously by food and oxygen, follows quantum physics laws. Chaos is the new science of non-linear mathematics and fractals. By measuring a few body parameters like blood pressure and blood sugar one cannot predict the future outcome in a human being, based on the outdated *laws of deterministic predictability*. The butterfly effect occurs in the human system almost always. Therefore, we have been "predicting the unpredictable".

Be that as it may, we have gone a step further by inventing chemical compounds to control some of these "abnormal" body parameters in healthy individuals. Long-term studies have shown this effort in very poor light. Time evolution in a dynamic system is such that the **probability** of a few abnormal parameters damaging the system in the long run is only fifty-fifty. A leading quantum physicist, Erwin Schrödinger, in his *Cat Hypothesis*, showed it elegantly.

Schrödinger hypothesized a closed box in which he put a live cat, a decaying atom with the half-life of half an hour, along with a phial of poison. In the deterministic predictability model when the atom decays and releases, say a proton, the latter would break the phial of poison to kill the cat. Unfortunately, the observer opening the box and looking in only could ascertain the future fate of the cat. The possibility of the cat dying was only fifty-fifty. The time of the atom decaying could not be predicted with certainty. Only the *Doctrine of Probabilities* of Blaise Pascal worked at the sub-atomic level of the quantum world. **So does the human body, strictly following the probability laws.** We are now back to square one. New thinking has to go into this field and medical science has to change for the better. The sooner the medical scientists realize this truth, the better for mankind. **The only certainty that works in the human body is uncertainty. The human body works as a whole. Reductionist science, which we follow at present, has no relevance to human physiology!**

The moral of the above story is that when one is healthy and does not have any kind of trouble (totally asymptomatic), one should try and follow the simple rules of living well. Those abnormal body parameters need not perturb one. Watchful expectancy with a change of mode of living would reverse the abnormality many a time. Doctors could help the hapless victims by reassuring him/her in such situations, in the absence of any positive findings on clinical examination and routine investigations. The doctor, however, should keep a careful watch for any new indications of trouble in the patient. This method pays rich dividends to the patient. If, on repeat examinations, the abnormality either gets worse or the patient starts getting symptoms, one could intervene at that stage without detriment to the final outcome.

You might wonder as to why a reader needs to know this much of physics? When one understands the basis of the interventions in medicine that the doctor advises, it is better for the patient to understand the implications of those interventions. Doctors also would do well to be acquainted with the scientific basis of their art to be able to guide their patients intelligibly. None of the medical interventions, including drug therapy, is without some danger lurking in the corner. **While there is no pill for every ill, in the long run, there certainly is an ill waiting to strike after every pill.** One, therefore, needs to weigh the pros and cons of those interventions to become an intelligible partner in one's own medical care. The days of doctors being paternalistic in management without taking the patient into confidence have gone. Today medicine has become a business and the consumer, the patient, has to be an informed customer lest he/she should be led up the garden path to the misty world of hi-tech medicine. One example would suffice.

If a middle aged man, in very good health and totally asymptomatic, goes for a check up, there is a possibility that the doctor might detect some elevation in his blood pressure. If the man happens to be a hypochondriac, this elevation could be very significant. I have even seen pressures of the order of 190/120 etc., in such situations that have come down to normal with tender loving care. In my opinion there is no entity called idiopathic primary hypertension. This diagnosis actually has some emotional and/or psychological cause for the raised pressure, which could be unraveled only by a placebo doctor who talks with patients and, does not talk to patients in a hurry. If there is no evidence of any other abnormality either on complete clinical examination, including the eyes, or in all the blood parameters, **the chances of that apparent elevation of blood pressure damaging the individual in the long run is only fifty-fifty. If that individual is put on antihypertensive drugs there is a fifty per cent chance that the drug is not needed as the pressure might come back to normal in the course of time. The other probability is that fifty per cent of the time the drug could damage the patient's health. No one could know in advance which fifty per cent works in which patient!**

By understanding the intricacies of the science of medicine, the doctor and his patient could understand the dangers of treatment as well as the benefits claimed by the drug companies. They could balance the risk-benefit ratio properly to be sensible partners in the treatment plans. **No doctor could be certain of what happens to the patient (with any disease) in the future with or without treatment. The risks and dangers of non-treatment strategy are only probabilities.** Prospective studies done recently, of cancer of the prostate with or without surgery, have hown that, in the long run, those who followed a watchful waiting strategy, instead of undergoing early surgery, did much better than those who had early surgery! Hypertension treatment, with any drug, in the long run, has been shown to have resulted in higher deaths in those treated compared to their normotensive cousins in society. This is the reason why the reader should understand the scientific basis of medicine.

> **One of the essential qualities of a clinician is interest in humanity, for the secret of the care of the patient is in caring for the patient.**
>
> —*Francis Weld Peabody (1881–1927)*

FURTHER READING

- Hegde BM. To do or not to do-Doctor's dilemma. *Kuwait Med J* 2001; 33(2): 107–110
- Firth WJ. Chaos-Predicting the unpredictable. *BMJ* 1991; 303: 1565–1568.
- Editor. *Cecil's textbook of Med ine* 2002 21st Edition. Page 1202.
- Hully S, Grady D, Bush T et al. Randomized trial of oestrogen plus progestin for secondary prevention of coronary heart disease in post-menopausal women. *JAMA* 1998; 280 605–613
- McCormack J and Greenhalgh T. Seeing what you want to see in randomized controlled trials: versions and perversions of UKPDS data. *BMJ* 2000; 320: 1720–23.
- Krumholz HM. Cardiac procedures, outcomes, and accountability. *N Engl J Med* 1997; 336: 1522–23.
- Angell M. Is academic medicine for sale? *N Engl J Med* 2000; 342: 1516–8.
- Editorial. Drug Company influence on medical education in USA. *Lancet* 2000; 356: 781–83.
- Gribbin J. *In search of Schrodinger's cat*. 1991. Transworld Publishers, 61-63, Uxbridge Road, London W5 5 SA.
- Hegde BM, Shetty MA, and Shetty MR. *Hypertension–Assorted Topics Book*. 1997. Bharathiya Vidya Bhavan, Bombay.
- Holmberg L, Bill-Axelson A, Helgesen F et al. A randomised trial comparing radical prostatectomy with watchful waiting in early prostate cancer. *N Eng Med J* 2002; 347: 781–89.
- Andersson OK, Almgren T, Persson B et al. Survival in treated hypertension: follow up after two decades. *BMJ* 1998; 317: 167–171.

CHAPTER 22

Ultra-Science

Progress is looking at the same thing from different angles. If we keep looking at something with the same angle that our forefathers were looking at, without questioning them at all, we would never progress. Change is progress and science is change.

"Shake a tree full of theorists, and twenty ideas will fall out" says Adam Riess of the Space Telescope Science Institute in Baltimore, USA. Albert Einstein's general and special relativity theories made the astonishing assertion that time, space and matter could be squeezed and stretched like India rubber. But he might have been a bit too hasty. Some sort of anti-gravity force—the "dark energy" (Einstein's cosmological term)—was needed to make his mathematical formulae work. He was greatly *relieved* in the 1920s when the theory of expanding Universe was formulated which would prove him right. But the present data from the Hubble's telescope has shown that while the Universe is expanding, it is moving in one direction faster than the rate of its expansion. There seems to be "something outside" pushing the Universe. This would prove Einsten wrong. The people working on this theory might get a Nobel for proving Einstein wrong. The new discovery now has almost confirmed the presence of the "dark energy" as real. Astronomers however would like to see a few more distant supernovas just to be sure, though.

"Recently, scientists made a powerful case that Einstein's blunder may actually have been another Nobel-worthy prediction," wrote Michael Lemonick in the *Times London* on April 16, 1980. "Tens and billions of years from now, our Milky Way galaxy will find itself alone in empty space with its nearest neighbours too far away to see. In the end, the stars will simply wink out and the Universe will end not with a bang but with the meekest of whimpers", he wrote.

Let us allow people to think freely and not restrict their thinking by our rigid narrow views of science. Condemning anything that does not fit in with our tunnel vision is not right. Wisdom does not belong to scientists only! Some thinking would, per force, be wrong. That does not mean that we should not let people think at all. That would be throwing the bath water out of the window with the baby inside.

Some one wrote the correct history of medicine thus: (author not known)

- 2000 BC—Here, eat this **root**.
- 1000 AD—That root is heathen, say this prayer.
- 1850 AD—That prayer is superstition. Here, drink this potion.
- 1940 AD—That potion is snake oil. Here, swallow this pill.
- 1985 AD—That pill is ineffective. Here, take this antibiotic.
- 2000 AD—That antibiotic is dangerous. Here, eat this **root**.

More and more scientists are realizing the futility of reductionist science. Dr Mariette Gerber of the National Institute of Medical Research in France, believes that such research methods, which attempt to isolate and examine the effects of a specific nutrient, are too narrowly focussed. In particular, single-agent studies may miss synergistic effects whereby different nutrients interact to lend increased disease fighting benefits. "**There is no guarantee that a nutrient like vitamin C exhibits the same behaviour when consumed alone as it may when consumed as a tomato**", wrote Mariette Gerber. The report from her institute issued in June 2001 states that "Wholistsic approach to research may provide new insights into science." *I have been writing about this for decades but no one took note. Instead, they ridiculed me! I am sure they would now sit up and take note now that it has come out in the World Cancer Research Journal.*

The core principle of Ayurveda is to have a wholistic look at the human body and mind to understand human diseases and to manage them. People trying to isolate alkaloids in Ayurvedic herbal medicines will have to be disappointed in the long run. There is a lot more in this universe than what meets the reductionist scientists' eyes and tools. The following studies would throw a lot more light on what I have been writing and saying so far. I hope deeper thinking and holistic research would unravel many more mysteries of this universe.

Coronary heart disease, claimed to be the ace killer in this century, was linked to lifestyle risk factors as smoking, high-fat diet, sedentary habits and non-adherence to medical advice. These have had multi-billion dollar business built around them in the last five decades. There have, however, been pointers even as far back as the 1950s that certain behaviour patterns might have a bearing on its incidence too. The latter was mostly swept under the carpet, as it did not generate business dollars!

A wealth of well-designed animal and human studies now have shown the direct link between behaviour and coronary disease. **The notable feature is that these behavioural factors predict future coronary heart disease events independently of the influence of lifestyle risk factors that are made much of. They are:**

- Hostility and anger (*Psychol Bull* 1996; 119: 322–348)
- Lack of social support (*Psychol Bull* 1996; 119: 488–531)
- Depression (*Circulation* 1995; 91: 999–1005)
- Low socioeconomic status with anxiety (*Circulation*; 99: 2192–2217)

Future interventions should concentrate on these factors more than all the lifestyle risk factors being sold to the gullible public. Two new studies **ENRICHD** and **SADHART** are looking into this and their results could alter our management strategies in coronary heart disease.

Newer studies have shown that atherosclerotic blocks (blocks seen in the angiograms) get worse with job stress (*BMJ* 1997; 314: 553–558). Psychosocial factors adversely affect the coronary arteries (Circulation 1995; 92:1720–1725). Episodes of acute anger could bring on a heart attack (*J Am Coll Cardiol* 2000; 36: 1781–1788). In patients with coronary disease and hostile personality, episodes of anger could bring on left ventricular dysfunction and heart failure (*J Am Coll Cardiol* 1993; 22: 440–448). Similarly, in everyday life, intense anger and stressful mental activities could provoke anginal pain and even infarct (*J Am Coll Cardiol* 1996; 27: 585–592). **Hostility has been discovered to be the "toxic" factor in human behaviour; it has several components such as aggressive and irritable feelings about others, and hostile thoughts about others. A recent meta-analysis revealed that hostility potential was the best predictor of all cause mortality!** (*Arch Intern Med* 1996; 156: 745–752)

Coupled with this is the data emerging from many new studies to show how time-honoured interventions like **prayer** could be of use in sickness. I am sure our "scientists" would be terribly angry at these studies! But remember that anger is the worst risk factor for coronary heart disease, as shown above in many elegant *scientific* studies. William Harris and his colleagues at the Mid American Heart Institute and the University of California in San Diego have shown, in an elegant *randomized, controlled, prospective study with impeccable study design,* that "remote, intercessory (praying for others) prayer was associated with lower Coronary Care Unit scores. These results suggest that prayer might be employed as an adjunct with significant benefit in the management of heart attack patients in the acute stage (*Arch Intern Med* 1999; 159: 2273–2278).

Many of the newer technologies, much touted, have been shown to be ineffective, if not dangerous, on long-term audits. Many drugs have been either proved ineffective or dangerous and have been withdrawn in the last couple of decades. Most of the fault lies in the methods of reductionist science applied to a dynamic system like the human body. The same holds good for other sciences like physics and chemistry.

The earlier report about vitamin C and tomato is a good example to show how the *whole* need not (usually is not) be the sum total of the *bits.* Nothing, in my opinion, that is complicated, becomes less complicated when looked at more carefully. On the contrary, new angle of research would bring out hidden facets of the mystery. Progress could, therefore, come from an open mind. Closed minds have no place in serious science. The new Indo-European etymological root of the word science is *skei,* which simply means *to cut into.* I feel that the only genuine scientist is an innocent child that explores anything given to it. Grown up scientists, who could keep a child's heart in their adulthood, would be wonderful scientists too! Otherwise, science would go after money and prestige, although many claim that scientists do what they do for the passion. Passion makes some of the best observations, but might draw, at times, wretched conclusions.

Money was the driving force in the reductionist sciences even from the very beginning. A glance at the early history of chemistry would show how! Alchemy was the forerunner of the modern chemistry and the former was used to fool all people all the time or to make it big by turning base metals into gold! However, chemistry could go back to its origin in the Khimi region (the land of black earth) on the Nile Delta some 4000 years ago. The first discovery was the finding that minerals when heated could result in the isolation of metals and glasses with useful properties. Those could be sold for profit! This science of chemistry spread gradually from the Arab world to Asia—gaining en route the secrets of gunpowder manufacture from the Chinese. Gunpowder did make lots and lots of money. The foundation of the Nobel Prize owes its existence to gunpowder, right?

I strongly feel that more than the outwardly, intellect-based, objective education, a good scientist needs inwardly, intuition-based, subjective education as well. The two together, in a balanced fashion, could bring forth real good scientists in the future, who have their own minds rather than the borrowed minds that cannot look at the same object from different angles. Science, like any other human endeavour, should be for the good of humankind. It should make man love man.

FURTHER READING

- Peter Medawar. *Limits to Science.*

CHAPTER 23

Problems in the Evidence of Evidence-Based Medicine

The oft repeated statement that the incidence of coronary artery disease is going up exponentially in the immigrant population (as also in others) needs further scrutiny. Is it just a statistical anomaly or a real increase, needs to be seen? In our reductionist biomedical model of diseases we use coronary artery blocks and coronary artery disease synonymously. Many people could have blocks in the epicardial vessels without any evidence of coronary artery disease, elegantly shown in the studies of Vietnam and Korean War casualties! Many of those that have innocent blocks could be provoked to have coronary artery disease by our precocious labeling them. Evidence based medicine cannot assess the gravity of frightening patients about fatal diseases and doctors predicting their unpredictable future course. Many of these youngsters could eventually suffer the ravages of the Ulysses syndrome.

Evidence-based medicine (EBM) has been defined as the "conscientious, explicit, and judicious use of current best evidence in making decisions about the care of individual patients. The practice of evidence-based medicine means integrating individual clinical expertise with the best available external clinical evidence from systematic research." More specifically, EBM reflects a concerted effort to systematically retrieve and synthesize data, make the data available to physicians, and incorporate it into practice. "Intuition and individual clinical experience are deemphasized and decision-making based on evidence is stressed. Although there have been some concerns about whether there is sufficient evidence to guide many of our clinical decisions, about what represents the best available evidence, and about the authoritarian voices of the EBM movement, it should be our goal to make the most informed medical decisions on behalf of patients", writes Howard Bauchner.

If one were to take a holistic view of coronary artery disease incidence one has to give equal weightage to the environment in which the immigrants are placed—their acculturation. Going to a foreign land in search of greener pastures, in itself, has the in-built anxiety factor that has a very great causal effect on their health status. With newer studies showing the mind as the major player in the causation of coronary artery disease, one wonders why the authors are still harping only on the time-honoured "risk factor hypotheses" of fat, blood pressure, diabetes etc. The latter could all be the genetic clusters in such individuals rather than being the cause of one another! The conventional fat hypothesis has led to the burgeoning business in anti-cholesterol drugs that seems to have only changed the label in the death certificates without changing the date! Too much drugging for lowering patient's blood sugar and blood pressure have both been counterproductive to say the least.

The family background of the immigrants and their economic status could also be contributing to the incidence of coronary disease. Coronary artery disease also follows the rule that poverty is the mother of most ills. Barker's hypothesis could be working in those immigrants that were born to abject poverty. Therefore, if future studies are being planned to study the reasons why the immigrants have precocious coronary disease the above mentioned suggestions could be incorporated there to make it more evidence based and authentic. We seem to be absolutely certain about the risk factors in coronary disease as we know very little about its causation. "Man is absolutely certain when he knows very little, with knowledge doubts increase", said Goethe.

Recent evidence points to the role of lifestyle modifications with a special stress on tranquility of mind as the best insurance against precocious coronary disease as also in the management of established CAD. That needs to be incorporated in the evidence-based management strategies of CAD.

FURTHER READING

- Stehbens WE. An appraisal of the epidemic rise of coronary heart disease and its decline. *The Lancet* 1987;182: 399–405.
- Enos WF, Holmes RH, Beyer J. Coronary artery blocks among US soldiers killed in action in Korea. *JAMA* 1953; 152: 1090–1093.
- Rang M. The Ulysses Syndrome, *Can Med Assn J* 1972; 106: 122–123.
- Bauchner H. Cumulative meta-analysis of therapeutic trials for myocardial infarction. *N Engl J Med* 1992; 327: 248–254.

What Doctors Don't Get to Study in Medical School

- Rozanski A, Blurnenthal JA, Davidson KW et al. The epidemiology, pathophysiology and management of heart diseases-milestones in cardiac prevention. *J Am Coll Cardiol* 2005; 45: 637–651.
- Hegde BM. Need for a change in medical paradigm. *Proc Royal Coll Physi Edin.* 1993; 23: 9–12.
- Jacobs D, Balckburn H, Higgins M et al. Report of a conference on low cholesterol and mortality association. *Circulation* 1992; 86: 1046–60.
- Sheppard J, Cobbe SM, Islers CG et al. Prevention of coronary artery disease. *N Engl J Med* 1995; 333: 1301–1307.
- Dunder K, Lind L, Zethelius B, et al. Increase in blood glucose concentration during antihypertensive treatment as a predictor of myocardial infarct. *BMJ* 2003; 326: 681.
- McCormack J, Greenhalgh T. Seeing what you want to see in research-The UPSPD study. *BMJ* 2000; 320: 1720–1723.
- Superko HR, Wood PD, Haskell WL. Coronary heart disease and risk factor modification: is there a threshold? *Am J Med* 1985: 78 826–38.
- Blumenthal J, M Babyak, et al. "Usefulness of psychosocial treatment of mental stress-induced myocardial ischemia in men." *American Journal of Cardiology*, 2002, Vol. 89. 164–168.
- Ornish D, Scherwitz LW, et al. "Intensive Lifestyle Changes for Reversal of Coronary Heart Disease." *Journal of the American Medical Association (JAMA)*, 1998, Vol. 280. 2001–2007
- Brody, Jane and Denise Grady, *The New York Times Guide to Alternative Health*. New York: New York Times Co., 2001. 203–244.

CHAPTER 24

Nanotechnology

Medical profession needs to have an idea as to what nanotechnology is all about and how nanotechnology could help us to preserve the health of the public. Nano-science, which threatens to change the way we practise modern medicine, is itself in a flux. The business community would want us to believe that nanotechnology would solve all our problems ranging from energy crisis, heart disease, drug manufacture, disease prevention, to cancer management. Richard Smalley, a Nobel Laureate chemist, had this to say in concluding the now famous Drexler-Smalley debate of the 1990s: "You and people around you have scared our children. I don't expect you to stop, but I hope others in the chemical community will join with me in turning on the light, and showing our children that, while our future in the real world will be challenging and there are real risks, there will be no such monster as the self-replicating mechanical nanobot of your dreams." To which Drexler, the Chairman of the Foresight Institute, responds by quoting Smalley on an earlier occasion. Smalley is reported to have said that if a scientist says that something is possible, he/she is probably underestimating the time it will take to fructify; but if a scientist says that something is not possible, he/she is wrong. It is no wonder that most people in the medical field know very little about nano-science.

Nanotechnology, a method primarily of molecular manufacturing, for the creation of tools, materials and machines that might eventually enable us to "snap together the fundamental building blocks of Nature easily, inexpensively, and in most of the ways permitted by the laws of Physics. One of the brilliant scientists, who is now the Evan Pugh Professor of Solid State and Emeritus Professor at the Pennsylvania State University, Rustum

Roy, is the real pioneering father of nanotechnology. Even at his age (80+) he has the enthusiasm of youth and continues to do research with the same passion.

Given the present gross exaggerations associated with the halo-word nano, I must confess that it was Rustom Roy in the early 50s, working as a chemist and now for well over sixty years, has worked with ions, atoms or molecules—all genuinely nano. By 1950 he had designed the *sol-gel* process, still the most widely used route to produce, relatively effortlessly, nanoparticles of myriad compositions. Using this route he and his team started to make genuine nanocomposites by the late eighties. By 1991, long before anyone else in the field, he convened a Symposium on Nanoscience and Technology at the Materials Research Society.

"The idea caught on; the salability of a euphonious slightly mysterious term became caught up in the corridors of Science Funding and the rest is (bad) history" he says with nostalgia. "Today, nanotechnology is a PR bonanza for a subset of science. It is focus of attention on nano, the very small, which had NEVER been neglected by chemists or biologists. Regrettably it causes the neglect of many other fields closer to society's needs– health of the masses, the environment, employment etc. –which are at the Giga end of the spectrum", opines Rustom Roy in one of his pensive moods.

In matters of inorganic chemistry and social activism Rustom was probably Linus Pauling's closest disciple. By chance he also worked with both Ivan Illich (of Medical Nemesis fame) and Norman Cousins, and thus was well schooled in the failures of conventional high-tech medicine.

Those fortuitous connections are what started Rustom Roy down the path of a scientific appraisal of the field. Moreover as an experimental scientist – Penn State's Materials Research Laboratory, which he founded, was ranked #1 in the world, by ISI, strictly on the strength of its Faraday like empirical experiment-based advances – Rustom Roy immediately grasped the value of masses of empirical data contained in long traditions of healing and went into scientifically validating them. And, most important of all, Rustom had his continuous, very successful research in the hard sciences not dependent on the medical establishment he was soon criticizing.

Rustom Roy, having been convinced of the futility of pursuing nanotechnology to cure all our ills, put together an unusual seminar on WHOLE PERSON HEALING (other end of nano-world) during the week ending 14th through 17th of April 2005 in Washington DC, which was a run away success. Now that Rustom Roy and Nobel Laureate Richard Smalley give credibility to this idea, let us come out of our delusion that genetic engineering and nanotechnology would solve all our problems, especially of poverty. Poverty is maintained in the world thanks to the rich man's proclivity for comfort and his greed.

World poverty is of gigantic proportions! Nearly 1.2 billion people live on less than $1 per day. More than a billion people do not get clean drinking water. More than 2 billion do not have access to any kind of sanitation. Nearly 1.5 billion people, mostly in larger cities in the third world breathe such polluted air that equals smoking three packets of cigarettes per day. Marine life exploitation, soil erosion, and water scarcity have reached the breaking point. Deforestation goes on unabated all over the world thanks to the greedy loggers. World population is going up by nearly 80 million per year. This could only be helped marginally if nanotechnology could produce cheap alternate energy sources in place of the fossil fuel. India, the largest democracy, is paying millions of dollars every year for fossil fuel.

If that money could be diverted to health care (clean drinking water for everyone, three square uncontaminated meals, a toilet for every house to avoid the ravages of hookworms, and avoidance of cooking smoke coming into the house with deadly carbon monoxide, and economic empowerment and education of women) world health scenario will change dramatically. Instead, if we concentrate on cancer treatment using nanotechnology and other treatment modalities we will, probably, end up with more problems than solutions.

There are so many imponderables in human physiology that one could never predict time evolution in human beings. The slight changes that we have the power to make in the initial state (like surgery in healthy people and genetically engineered molecules introduced into the body) using our hi-tech stuff might not do what they are intended to do, as time evolves. On the contrary, they might even harm (they have) as time evolves through the "butterfly effect" of Edward Lorenz.

Cancer has remained undefeated so far! Nano effort cannot change that so easily. War on cancer has to be fought on a holistic front. While the theoretical possibilities of nanoscience look endless with scientist turned businessmen like Drexler making us believe that the day is not far off when they could even manufacture self replicating nanobots in place of the robots of today. Nanobots could roam the world producing their "kids" at their own sweet will! Science always tried to unravel the mysteries of the universe. When science tries to control the natural laws of the universe, nature would certainly revolt!

FURTHER READING

- Michael Wilson (editor) et al. *Nanotechnology: Basic Science and Emerging Technologies*, CRC Press 2002
- Michael Gross. *Travels to the Nanoworld: Miniature Machinery in Nature and Technology*, Perseus Publishing, 2001.
- Drexler-Smalley Debate. *Chemical Engineering News*. 2003; 81: December 1st issue.
- Roy R. Personal Communications. 2005
- Wolf EL. *Nanophysics and Nanotechnology: An Introduction to Modern Concepts in Nanoscience*, Wiley-VCH, 2004.
- Hegde BM. Clinician's view of whole person Healing. *Procs Whole Person Healing Summit*, Washington DC April 14–17, 2005.
- Jones RAL. *Soft Machines - Nanotechnology and Life*, OUP, 2004.
- Hegde BM. Chaos- a new concept in science. *J Assoc Physi India* 1996; 44: 167–68.
- Rietman Ed, et al. Molecular Engineering of Nanosystems, Springer Verlag, 2001.
- Turton R. *The Quantum Dot: A Journey into the Future of Microelectronics*, Oxford University Press, 1999.
- Drexler E. *Engines of Creation: The Coming Era of Nanotechnology*, Anchor, 1987.

CHAPTER 25

Modern Medical Research- Time is Ripe for its Audit

> Two roads diverged in the woods and I-
> Took the one less traveled by,
> And that has made all the difference.
> —Robert Frost

Modern medicine abounds in mostly repetitive research. Original articles on research findings pour into the literature at a phenomenal speed of 7% per month. In addition, we have web sites for free publication. In peer-reviewed journals, by and large, only positive research is published although there are a few exceptions. Publication bias is not totally eliminated. Consequently, all that is published is not necessarily true! One or two reputed journals require the authors to give the details of funding for research. At times, it becomes difficult to unravel the hidden agenda behind these studies.

It is estimated that there are more than 40,000 biomedical journals as of now. Inducements for publishing the desired results have ranged from large sums of money to entertain at international conferences in five-star hotels to other perks while the work is in progress s(Looking the Gift horse in the mouth, *JAMA,* 1999 April). The researchers are looking primarily for p-values, confidence intervals, and statistical significance in the routine IMRDC presentation. A few complicated charts and diagrams make for the best presentation and would be acceptable to editors and reviewers. The status of the institution where the research work is done matters a lot, if not to the reviewers in the blinded review system, at least to the editorial team.

Conference presentation of data is in no way better. The speaker flashes slides with complicated statistical data and a lot of numbers on each slide, which remain, on the screen for a very short time because of time constraints. The audience gets hardly any time to grasp the data, leave alone critically evaluating the same. By the time the listener gets to see the data properly the slide has already changed. With all the social functions there is hardly any time left for question-answer session at the end of each presentation. There are other seasoned keynote speakers who are past masters in the trade of feeding dubious data in the most fashionable way with the help of modern gadgetry and funding from pharmaceutical giants.

Let us look at some of the recent publications. There was a report on zinc supplementation in childhood to reduce morbidity and mortality due to diarrhoeal diseases and pneumonia. In addition, zinc is supposed to help growth in the poor children on inadequate diets. The studies were done mainly in third world countries. The meta-analysis showed that zinc supplementation is very important (*BMJ* 1999; 319: 1521). Sure enough the drug companies must be ready with zinc in various forms at exorbitant prices in the market!

One of these studies was done in a remote village in rural India, and the same investigator has now got lots of dollars extra grant to repeat the study in Africa. The original researchers and the funding came from one of the most prestigious institutions in the West. Of course, we have enough of their collaborators here. **Nearly one thousand very poor children, mostly from the slums, were picked up for the study. The following rules were strictly followed:**

- The children or their parents did not know that they were participating in a drug trial.
- No attempt was ever made to either educate them on preventive measures or change their unhealthy environment.
- Their diet remained what it was before the study, except in one half zinc supplements were added.
- They continued to drink water from an open canal, which was stagnant most of the time with very little rainfall in that part of the country.
- This water is definitely unfit even for animals in the West.
- The mortality and morbidity were recorded scientifically most faithfully!

The special clinic set up during the study period meticulously did the work as per the protocol, unconcerned about the other medical needs of the community, only to close shop after the work got over. This is pure exploitation of hapless human beings in the name of research! I wonder how many such inhuman and criminal acts are swept under the carpet to get research data! **We have organizations to question animal experiments even in our country, but alas, there are no such organizations to question misuse of hapless human beings.** No wonder Britain has a Royal Society for Prevention of Cruelty to Animals but only a National Society for Children. Is it because man hates man that he has suddenly started loving animals? May be it is because animals do not have the power to protest, but these unfortunate ignorant villagers are being treated worse than dumb animals.

The reader would have by now got an idea of the impact of this study. The primary aim of the study was to prove the hypothesis that zinc, a micronutrient, added to food could make all the difference. During the study the hapless children continued to die or suffer the consequences of infective diarrhoea and pneumonia in their own setting.

If the same dollars were to be used to supply clean drinking water and also to educate the poor people in hygienic methods, diseases would have vanished without any zinc! One could have eradicated infective diarrhoea in that part of the country and people would have enjoyed clean water supply forever. In addition, they could have been empowered with the knowledge to prevent diseases.

Reductionist science, looking at bits and pieces, has already done enough damage by way of wrong conclusions drawn from such studies that do not look at the organism as a whole in its environment. However, reductionist science has been a very good business proposition. Would they dare do such studies in the West? Does this not amount to exploiting the poor?

Let us look at some of the other happenings in this field. Recent studies in Britain once again reaffirmed my belief that poverty (may be even relative) is the basic problem in illness (*BMJ* 1999;314:1522). This is more glaring in the Indian scenario. The poor pay for their poverty with their lives.

In the United States alone there have been more than 1,00,000 mistakes by doctors ranging from minor faults to major accidents like amputating the wrong leg! Nearly 8000 mistakes, including many deaths, were due to wrong drug combinations. Majority of them were due to the bad handwriting of doctors and a few were, of course, the mistakes of pharmacists. One could imagine the gravity of the situation elsewhere. The time has come to be open about this and teach medical students that mistakes are inevitable and they should try to minimize them. When they occur it is better to take the patient and relatives into confidence and explain the human aspect of medicine. Secrecy now, leads to trouble later (*BMJ* 1999;314:1519).

Crime is no stranger to medical science either. "Man, whether in the palace or pad, castle or cottage is governed by the same emotions and passions," wrote Shakespeare years ago. We have to humanize medicine a lot. With the advent of modern hi-tech gadgets doctors might get an idea that they are omnipotent and they could do anything from conception to death. The truth is that man's capacity to run this world with only free will has not been proven as yet. The twentieth century has definitely proved one important thing and that is the enormity of man's ignorance. But there are doctors who still feel that they could do anything and get away with it. One pathologist in a children's' hospital in England has a collection of 2000 hearts and 800 other organs of children collected after postmortem examinations between 1988 and 1995, without the consent of either the parents or the authorities. The innocent parents were told that their dead babies were all intact and only bits of tissues were taken for further examination. A thorough enquiry has been ordered (*BMJ* 199;314:1518).

Many times in the past I have written, and have been badly rebuked by my peers for this, that money and its effect on the human mind could have deleterious effects on our patients in any corporate hospital set up! "Money," said John Kenneth Galbraith in his celebrated book *The Age of Uncertainty*, "is a singular thing. It ranks with love as man's greatest source of joy and with death as his greatest source of anxiety." Now we have scientific proof that patients who undergo kidney dialysis in a "hospital for profit" set-up suffer more than in a teaching set-up. In the USA, on an average, about 2,00,000 patients undergo dialysis every year and about 67% of them do so in the "hospital for profit" set-up. These are the ones who have more complications and have less opportunity for transplants. The mind set of doctors in those set-ups is that if patients continue to get dialyzed it is more profitable for the hospital rather than sending the patient for transplant. Also, the patient has more complications and the profit goes up with more interventions! (*New Engl J Med* 1999; 341: 1653–1691)

In contrast, purely governmental set-ups give their patients a raw deal. This was shown by the inferior quality of treatment given to cancer patients in NHS hospitals in the UK (*BMJ* 199;319:1521). The NHS is suffering from lack of funds very badly. That brings us to the dire need for doctors to be aware of the enormous strengths and also weaknesses of the complementary medicines, which could ease this malady to a great extent. This is now realized in the UK where students are given instructions on complementary theory (*BMJ* 199;319:1561). **While I have been advocating that for more than two decades my friends have been labeling me a quack of the refined variety!**

124   What Doctors Don't Get to Study in Medical School

Modern medicine is not all that safe and effective as it is made out to be. Every single advance in therapy with modern methods is fraught with the danger of unforeseen side effects. It is now known that the prohibitively expensive bone marrow transplants that are being advertised even in India are not safe in the long run. Long term survivors of bone marrow transplants have **four times higher chance of getting other cancers** as compared to their peers who did not have bone marrow transplants. (*Ann Intern Med* 1999; 131: 1738). It may be that they do not live long enough to experience this! Adverse Drug Reactions have been the fourth-most important cause of death in America, the third being hospitals and doctors (*JAMA* 2000; 284: 483–485).

"Prediction is difficult, especially of the future," wrote Neils Bohr, a Nobel Laureate. Human beings are immeasurably more complex than any system in this Universe. It is impossible to predict who will contract which disease, or who will respond to which treatment. Both of these are intrinsic and not necessarily due to either absence of any routine check up or other precautions. Time and again this has been brought out by studies. A recent one is the routine screening for small vessel abnormality, called aneurysm, inside the brain, and might bleed in those having a family history. This study showed that it is impossible to predict who would bleed even if screened. This is true of cancer of the prostate and many other (any other) illnesses (*BMJ* 1999; 319:1512).

Happiness is living dangerously but sensibly. Ayurveda has the following advice. If you have a good appetite, have regular bowel movements, a proper water works system, and you sleep well and have the enthusiasm to work, you only have to keep your mind free of all negative feelings like hatred, jealousy and pride and fill your mind with universal love, and you will live happily as long as you live. You will certainly not live here forever. What a beautiful advice given thousands of years ago! Live and let live by loving all creatures on the planet!

> I eat when I am hungry,
> I drink when I am thirsty,
> If heavens don't fall down,
> I shall certainly live till I die.
>
> —*Irish Proverb*

Further Reading

- John Abramson. *Overdo$ed America*. Harper Collins, 2004.

CHAPTER 26

Chaos – A New Science

Whereas all the theories in biology emphasized steady states and equilibrium, the new theory of Chaos deals with non-linearity, complexity, and randomness. The theory began sometime in early 1970s. Mathematicians, physicians, biologists and chemists were the ones interested in the beginning, but this is the theory that applies 100% to the human body. It is now placed in the same category as quantum physics. This new theory came up because of the realization by narrowly specialized scientists that it is impossible to predict the future accurately in any dynamic system. We doctors deal with one of the most complicated organisms: man. Therefore, an understanding of chaos theory is essential for all doctors.

All through the ages, biology has been using linear relationships in predicting the future. We have been predicting the unpredictable. Future prediction is difficult. The new science of chaos, completely based on non-linearity has shown that predictability is only an exception rather than a rule even in simple physical systems. To answer questions like "who will get a heart attack?" and "how long before this HIV-positive patient develops AIDS?" we could use non-linear mathematics. Non-linear systems can seek out and maintain essentially an optimum state in response to a wide variability of external conditions. "It is precisely this feature that gives us individuality and continuity."

In fact, there is indication that the normal heartbeat is irregular, indeed chaotic. It could easily be kicked from the normal state by electric current or other shock into a state of cardiac arrest, and with luck and skill, we may be able to kick it back again. Similarly, health is a chaotic fluctuating attraction, which co-exists alongside with the fixed attraction called "death" in a multidimensional-phase space, which we cannot try to measure. Illness, in some measure, is in between these two attractors. This is precisely the reason why doctors are not able to predict, based on the multitude of epidemiological studies, when a given patient will die of cancer, heart attack or what have you. More insights into this new theory should give us more important clues as to how a living organism, like man, can maintain himself in the ocean of "so-called" risks around us and indeed might even give us a clue as to how man exists at all on this planet in the first place.

To sum up, very many systems, when viewed in isolation, have an intrinsically unpredictable behaviour; but when looked at as a whole, give us a broader view, enabling us to predict more accurately. Most systems are inter-dependent, called "mode-locking"—they work in tandem. For example, in the human body, the two systems locked to one another are breathing and heart rhythm. Many other areas could be studied, such as epidemics like chickenpox and measles, the pattern of water dripping from a tap, blood sugar fluctuations, and moving fluctuations. Ovulation cycles, neuronal discharges, and cardiac arrhythmias could be the most profitable areas of study in non-linear analysis.

Currently, our knowledge of many diseases and their therapy in biology is largely empirical, based on educated guesses under large doses of luck. Descriptive classification of all kinds of arrhythmias and their treatment—drug as well as cardioversion—is again based on luck. Applying non-linear equations to define particular arrhythmias could give us a much better insight into their treatment. We can even calculate the exact dose of electric current needed to bring an arrhythmia back to its healthy state.

We have been studying non-linearity and mode-locking in heart rate variability (HRV) for a number of years and the resulting papers appear in many journals. We have gone a step further compared to other workers in the field, in that we have discovered a new computer graphic model of the physiology, or otherwise of the heart's function, based on HRV: non-linearity of the conventional linear measures of the surface ECG like ST segment etc. They have been fine tuned by us using a complicated mathematical process – wavelet analysis quotient. This may be the beginning of a new era of understanding the complicated, hitherto ill-understood facet of human physiology.

FURTHER READING

- Firth WJ. Chaos. *BMJ* 1991: 303 :1565–1568
- Wagner CD, Nufz B, Persson PB. Chaos in blood pressure control. *Cardiovasc Res.* 1996; 31: 380–7.
- Gleik J. *Chaos – Making a new science book*. Cardinal, London, 1987
- Hegde BM. Chaos – a new concept in science. *J Assoc Physi India* 1996; 44: 167–68.

CHAPTER 27

Where is the Mind? Never Mind!

Philosophers, physicians, poets, thinkers, scientists, and, of course, lay men were equally perplexed about this enigma called the mind. What is the mind? Where is it? Most of them did feel the presence of their minds, though. Mind is like the wind, which the poet described thus:

> Who has seen the wind?
> Neither you, nor I,
> When the trees dance and bend,
> The wind is passing by!
>
> —*Christina*

That is true of the mind as well. People have been trying to fix the mind, like all other cellular structures of the human anatomy, to a particular organ. This organ-based medicine, like the modern so-called scientific medicine, used to believe that the mind resided in the heart, for a very long time. Words like sweet heart, hard hearted, kind hearted, large hearted, you are my heart etc., originated from that wrong impression. Physicians, led by the Canadian brain surgeon, Penfield, tried to locate the mind in some part of the brain. They did succeed temporarily though, as some of the bodily functions were controlled by certain parts of the brain, the latter being the headquarters of the central nervous system.

Brain, or for that matter, any other organ in the body, could not be the seat of the mind. The mind could never be thought of in terms of cellular structures. The human brain, for example, has billions of cells. A small grain of salt has more than ten billion atoms. If the cells of the brain were to be the seat of the mind, the latter would not be in a position even to comprehend a small grain of salt, leave alone this vast Universe. The science of Robotics, which is nearly seventy years old, has not been able to replicate the human mind to be packed inside a human robot. The future science of nanotechnology which predicts that it could create self replicating nanobots would also meet with the same fate. Richard Smalley, a Nobel Laureate chemist, wrote to the father of the nanobot hypothesis, Eric Drexler, a young PhD from MIT, who has already started a new company, Foresight Inc, to manufacture and sell these nanobots, that "his ideas would never see the light of the day in the foreseeable future anyway."

Sending a man to the moon is a child's play compared to mimicking the comprehension and enjoyment of the vast blue sky with its rainbow, by the human mind. It would have been a greater scientific feat if we could succeed in sending man, with a smile on his face, to his neighbor's drawing room to have a cup of tea there. Enjoying Nature's beauty and loving thy neighbor are both functions of the human mind, which baffles ordinary mortals, including that privileged class called scientists.

New wisdom seems to be dawning on science, which now has changed its etymology from that of *knowledge* to the new Sanskrit root *skei*—cut into. When you keep cutting the cell into bits and pieces to get at the atoms and beyond, you feel the mind. Oppenheimer (American), Enrico Fermi (Italian), and Neils Bohr (Scandinavian) together tried to split the atom into smaller particles called hydrons. Their teacher, a Nobel Laureate physicist, Max Bohm, a very wise scientist that he was, had warned them that *"this little atom which they were attempting to split would certainly teach mankind a lesson or two."* **This proved to be prophetic.** Mankind is not only suffering from the atomic fallouts in every sphere of human life on this planet, but we do not even know what to do with the deadly *plutonium waste*, which has a half-life of five hundred years! Our future generations could hold us responsible for this *"mindless"* action of ours.

Take time to watch the word, mindlessness! Indian ancient **rishis** had prophesied thousands of years ago in the **Vedic** wisdom about this possibility. Modern science realized this only now that they have been able to split the hydrons further into the ***leptoquarks.*** The latter seem to be the same in all living and non-living things. They seem to be moving freely inside and outside of living things. But they are so small that they defy their study and definition. They could be comprehended by the mind, though. It is beautifully described in the **Upanishads:**

Bahiranthaschya Bhootaanaam, Charam Acharam evacha,
Sookshmavatheth avijneyam; doorastham cha anikethacha tat.

(It is both inside and outside of all living things—it is moving and could be stationary as well; it is so subtle that it could not be examined and understood, for those who are not aware of its existence it is very far; for those who know, it is very close!)

Physics of leptoquarks and Indian Upanishads have realized the unitary nature of all things on this planet. Western scientists are looking to the East for inspiration. **The mind is a subatomic quantum state (quantum physics deals with the subatomic world). Human mind, or otherwise called the human consciousness, is a quantum level thinking. Just as the "seed has the tree" in it, the zygote, that little speck of protein that man is on the day he is conceived inside his mother's womb, knows all about every other living thing in the Universe because there are no two living things having identical genetic make-up.** Modern science makes out four levels of consciousness—waking consciousness, the dreaming, the sleeping and the quantum consciousness. Similar classification was there in Indian wisdom for thousands of years! Shivam, sundaram, advaitham, and chathurtham were the four stages identical to the latest scientific consciousness.

Quantum physicists realized their mistake only after they could not fathom the nature of leptoquarks that their reductionist theories could only go that far and not beyond the quantum stage of matter. They also realized that at **the quantum level mind and matter were the same and it did not matter what you are talking about!** Einstein's arrogant hypothesis that "nothing could move faster than light" was quickly proved wrong. With the realization that mind and matter are but the same, the speed of mind at phenomenal rate could be comprehended. **"Manovega" (speed of the mind) was an ancient concept, which has been recently rediscovered by science, not invented! Teleportation is the new name of the game.**

Even in the past there were thinking scientists, but their voices were drowned in the more powerful voices of the reductionist **scientists. The latter science had money value and was a salable commodity.** The more sensible theories of uncertainty principle by Werner Heisenberg and the Cat theory of Schrödinger (Schrödinger's cat) were all but swept under the carpet. People could build bridges across rivers (but not between man and man), they could build sky scrapers, super highways, send rockets into space, and communicate with distant people through wireless means, and even could send man into space with the help of reductionsist science.

Powerful nations made their day with wars, born in the petty minds, resulting in human misery on a very large scale. The fallout of reductionist science has not been for holistic human development. To cap it, science has helped destroy the bounties of Nature; man is threatening to completely destroy Nature.

Is Science Bad?

Not at all! Science, in the correct sense, is the only saviour of mankind. Science could make man realize the secrets of Nature to see how he could use science for the good of humanity. It is the **mind of the scientist or his financial master that has created misery for mankind and never science by itself.** In fact, without a scientific temper man could sink himself into the valley of illogicalism. Otto Frisch and Rudolf Pearls were responsible for conceiving the formula for the first atom bomb. But it was the mind of Harry Truman and Winston Churchill that resulted in its being dropped on that fateful August morning in 1945 on Hiroshima resulting in instantaneous death of more than 80,000 people within minutes. Thousands have died since all over the world due to atomic weapons! **Culprit, then, is not science but the human mind.**

How Could we Change This?

Both Churchill and Truman were born with a mind with only two natural instincts, that of self-preservation and procreation, like Gautama Buddha, Mahaveera or Mahatma Gandhi. At that stage there was no difference at all. How did the minds of Hitler and his ilk become what they were? It was our training the innocent human mind of every child in the **bad ways of the world.** The latter include competition, one up-man ship, hatred, and jealousy, anger, pride, ego and super ego. These are the traits we have inherited from the so-called scientific temper of the reductionist science, where competition is the key word. In the new science of holism (non-linear and CHAOS science) one looks at the whole with love and co-operation. **With this realization, we should move fast to change the training systems in our primary schools where the seed of all the bad habits are sown in the innocent minds of our little tiny tots.**

If you ponder about how innocent children that they were, Churchill, Truman, and Hitler, became warmongers later in adulthood, you would quickly realize the impact of our educational system. One has only to look beyond one's nose to realize the folly of our modern educational system of competition, ranks, prizes, and what have you. This was known to our Indian ancient wisdom when the following was written to train the human mind into tranquility:

> **To work alone thou has the right,**
> **But never to the fruits thereof,**
> **Be thou not actuated by the fruits of action,**
> **Nor be thou attached to inaction.**
>
> **Oh Dhananjaya, abandoning attachment**
> **And regarding success and failure alike,**
> **Be steadfast in yoga; perform thy duties,**
> **Even-mindedness is called Yoga.**
>
> —*Bhagavad Gita*

The stress here is on **even-mindedness**. A friend of mine, who is very successful in the conventional sense of the word, asked me if this line of thinking were pursued could there be progress **in the world. Many in that company naturally agreed with him.** He is a very successful doctor in that city, if success could be assessed by the amount of money one makes and also the power that one wields! Unfortunately, all the progress today has only resulted in bringing misery to mankind. There is no peace anywhere. United States of America, which is very successful in that sense, is in the grip of teenage violence where high school students shoot one another. They are now doing a bit of introspection. The innocent children, after studying in the schools become criminals, aping their adults in society. Daily we suffer the subtle white-collar crime in the name of science and technology. The food we eat is almost poisonous. Today, Europe is reeling under the threat of American ban on their meat export because the meat is found to be badly poisoned due to various genetic engineering methods. Tobacco is killing millions.

Every single killer disease, starting from heart attack to cancer, is now thought to originate in the **human mind.** Their cure or otherwise also depends on the **mind. Every human cell, including the heart muscle cell or the cancer cell, has its subatomic mind that either makes or breaks the final outcome!** Short-term quick fixes to make money, like drugs and surgery, are only temporary palliation. Long-term gains by way of primordial prevention depend on the **mind, the even-mind of yoga!**

If I am able to make the reader realize **the gravity of the problem and dire need to change** the way we live, to have a tranquil mind as the cure for all human ills, I will have achieved some success. Even very successful people in the worldly sense did get better by their philanthropic acts and not by amassing more wealth. Rockefeller Foundation and Ford Foundation are the success stories of their founders who changed with the vision of an even mind. One could get worldly riches also with having an even mind. One does not have to compete with others to destroy them to build oneself. One could live and let live with co-operation as the motto. The new science of the mind and its quantum consciousness would be able to send man not only to the moon but also to the neighbour's house with a smile.

Love thy enemy, love thy neighbour.
—Jesus Christ

Are we not all same on this planet? How then could you compete with your brother? Co-operate with him and love him.

Allah Ho Akbar!
—Holy Quran

Where is the mind? Never mind—it is everywhere inside and outside! Do not search for it outside of you, having the same all over you in every cell of your body of which there are one hundred thousand billion in all.

FURTHER READING

- Frawley David. *Mind in Ayurveda.* Banarsidas Dasgupta, Benaras India 1993.

CHAPTER 28

Euboxic Medicine

Modern medicine, having had a great influence from the West, especially the USA, is slowing going away from the suffering patient to the laboratory, where most of the management decisions are taken. This is very unfortunate. The younger generation of doctors is brainwashed to think that if the laboratory reports are normal, the patient should be all right. On the contrary, when the reports are abnormal, the poor patient is either drugged, or operated upon, irrespective of whether he is suffering or not. The main thrust seems to be to get the reports right! In the computerization era, this boils down to having the right boxes in the case-sheet properly marked in the right places—the **euboxic state.** Even when the patient dies, the doctors seem to be happy, as long as the patient had an euboxic death, i.e., at the time of death all the test result boxes were correctly marked, mainly to save the doctor's skin.

This is very sad, indeed! Many times, even when the person is absolutely asymptomatic and fit, some report or the other, of which there could be hundreds today, on a routine check-up, might deviate from the accepted norms for a given laboratory. This is scientifically called the false positive report further discussed in detail in the next chapter. The false positive reports would result in the poor man being labeled a patient and dealt with accordingly. While trying to bring the test results back to the normal range, the hapless person might be robbed of his health and happiness. Sir George Pickering, Regius professor of medicine at the Oxford and Johns Hopkins Universities, had once said about drug treatment of asymptomatic mild–moderate high blood pressure patients: "the patient loses the rights enshrined in the preamble to the American Constitution written in 1772 by Thomas Jefferson, of *life, liberty, and pursuit of happiness."*

Antihypertensive drugs "may or may not change his longevity; liberty he hardly could have what with all the restrictions put on him, and happiness becomes a thing of the past," said Professor Pickering.

Here is an interesting personal anecdote. I once saw a young man of 37 who had been working in the Gulf with lots of anxiety. His family was back home in India—young wife and two small kids. The man became very anxious and failed to get sleep. He got into the habit of taking alcohol for sleep and became addicted to it. He started getting vague chest discomfort, which was, clinically, anything but cardiac in origin. He consulted a couple of doctors in Dubai who told him that he did not have any heart disease. They did not, however, bother to relieve him of his incapacitating symptoms.

When he came back to India, he saw a doctor in a big city, who got him completely checked up, including a coronary angiogram, thallium scanning, echocardiogram, stress test etc., in addition to all the available blood tests at that time. At the end of all that he was told that the pain was not from the heart, but was not told what the pain was due to, and how to get rid of the pain. An empathetic look at this hapless young man would convince a good doctor how badly depressed he was and, if one went into his mind, one could unravel the mysteries of his suffering. Clinical, patient-oriented medicine, could have easily given away the diagnosis without the loss of such hefty sums of money, to get his heart into the euboxic state. This kind of medical practice does nothing for the relief of the patient's suffering. But the whole process is now geared to get money for the establishment. Doctors are under severe pressure to perform or perish!

A recent study of diabetics, discovered by routine screening of the asymptomatic population, revealed that the meticulous control of blood sugar helped mainly those who were symptomatic to begin with, **and not those who had no symptoms!** Same logic holds good for coronary artery disease, where bypass surgery has become a fashion and a compulsion these days. Gullible public are told that **"blood is better than drugs"** in the management of coronary artery disease. The truth, however, is that only those patients with severe symptoms of chest pain and breathlessness, that get very good relief of their symptoms, allowing them to lead a near normal life, whereas the asymptomatic people with even advanced epicardial coronary artery blocks shown by the angiogram, get very little benefit, unless they have very poor heart function, again felt by the patient as incapacitating breathlessness.

The inner secret is very simple. While, at a given point in time, there could be a few million patients who have symptoms, there could be at the same time, billions who could be shown to have abnormal reports of some sort or the other. The latter is a better business proposition, either to sell drugs or to do surgical corrections. Even the tall talk about early screening to catch diseases 'young," has not borne fruit by the audits all over the world. This is graphically brought out in a recent editorial in the *British Medical Journal* under the caption *Screening could seriously damage your health.*

It was estimated, at one stage, that there could be about 50–60 million 'healthy' Americans, who have *white-coat hypertension* (Doctor induced blood pressure rise). If all of them were to be immediately put on drugs like the latest calcium channel blockers and ACE inhibitors, drug companies could easily net about eight billion dollars per year! Lowering elevated blood pressures of the type described above, rarely does any good to the person concerned, but could, rarely harm him! In the long run, drug treated hypertensives have 2–3 times higher death rate due to various causes, compared to their normotensive cousins, even when their pressures are adequately controlled to get them into the **euboxic state.**

Time evolution in a dynamic human system does not depend on a few phenotypic characteristics, like blood pressure and blood cholesterol or sugar, but depends on the total initial state of the organism. In addition, changing the initial state in any direction with drugs may not hold good to give better results over a period of time. Linear mathematics has very little to do with future predictions in human beings; non-linear mathematics is not being used in medicine, unfortunately.

Similar audit reports are appearing about cancer screening as well. Medical profession has enough on its plate if it cares to look after all the sick people in this world, and would, certainly, have no time to meddle with the apparently healthy in society. Even today, nearly 80% of the world's population does not have access to modern medicine. A recent BBC programme in London showed how the poor people in society still have the highest incidence of all diseases even in advanced countries, while the rich and the strong are healthier. The reasons alluded to are very simple. The rich these days have **healthier life styles compared to the poor.** The rich smoke less, eat more sensibly relying basically on fruits and vegetables, drink less or abstain, exercise more, and more than all that, have better incomes to be less anxious about their next meal. The last one is said to be the greatest distress for the poor. **Poverty has been shown to be the womb of all illnesses.**

The poor get ill because they have unhealthy lifestyles with more distress than the rich do, and the rich get illness because of the **fear of the less fortunate in society.** Recent studies in the USA have shown that this fear of the poor drug addicts and criminals is one of the main stressors for the rich in that country. As the gulf between the rich and the poor is widening, illness goes up on both sides of the fence. Those of us interested in the long-term solutions to man's ills, should economically empower the poor and teach them better lifestyles.

There are a couple of other myths to be demolished in modern medicine. **One is that it is the change in lifestyle and better food that has brought down the incidence of all diseases, and not the hi-tech modern drugs or surgery. The second is that human life span has not gone up a wee bit in the last hundred years. What has gone up, on the contrary, is "life expectancy", a statistical term, which could easily be confused to be synonymous with life span. It is not!** Genetic engineering tricks to increase life span have not succeeded so far; even if they do, one would not be able to halt senility. Those efforts might end up adding years to life but not life to those years!

Long live clinical medicine of doing most good to most people most of the time, following the Hippocratic code of "cure rarely, comfort mostly, but console always." Death and disease are two different entities and have very little in common. Death is inevitable, as of now. Modern medicine has not been able to postpone or avoid death, but it could make life tolerable if one lives sensibly. Trying to live forever is foolish even today, as it was during the time of Bernard Shaw. Euboxic medicine is not the answer to the ills of society, but human and humane medicine is the need of the hour. Let us pass on this message to the medical students when they are still young. Medicine should not be taken to the market place, where market forces distort scientific data to suit the business convenience. This was brought home so beautifully in a recent study published in the *Journal of the American Medical Association.*

Many of the imaginary epidemics of diseases are brought on by the medical profession to scare the common man! In an editorial *Do epidemiologists cause epidemics,* The Lancet brings out the truth. Let us, instead, concentrate on doing maximum good to the suffering humanity, dysboxic as they are, and try to bring their whole clinical condition to the euboxic state.

FURTHER READING

- Davidoff F. *Who has seen a blood sugar?* Book Ed. American College of Physicians, 1998.
- Hegde BM, Shetty MA, Shetty MR. *Hypertension-Assorted Topics.* Bhavan's Publications, Bombay, 1995.
- Goddijin PPM, Bilo HJG, Feskens EJM et al. Longitudinal study of glycaemic control and quality of life in patients with Type 2 diabetes mellitus referred for intensified control. *Diabetic Medicine* 1999;16:23-30.
- Hegde BM. Coronary artery disease-time for reappraisal. *Proc Royal Coll Physi Edin*. 1995;26:421-24.
- Krumholz HM. Cardiac procedures, outcomes, and accountability. *N Engl J Med* 1997;336:1522-23.
- Stewart-Brown S & Farmer A. Screening could seriously damage your health. *BMJ* 1997;314:533.
- Firth WJ. Chaos-predicting the unpredictable. *BMJ* 1991; 303: 1565-68.
- Selly S, Donovan J, Faulkner A, Coast J, Gillatt D. *Diagnosis, management, and screening of early localized prostate cancer-review*. Bristol: Health care Evaluation Unit. University of Bristol, 1996.
- Hegde BM. Medical Humanism. *Proc Royal Coll Physi Edin*. 1997; 27:65-67.
- Cambell EG, Louis CS,& Blumenthal D. Looking a gift horse in the mouth-corporate gifts supporting life sciences research. *JAMA* 1999;279:995-999.
- Editorial. Do epidemiologists cause epidemics? *Lancet* 1993;341:993-994.

CHAPTER 29

Evidence Based or Evidence Burdened Medicine?

Modern medicine, with all its hi-tech and claptrap, is still following the outdated linear mathematics. Human body is dynamic and is never linear. Continuously run by food and oxygen, the body follows only non-linear rules. Normality, defining normal human beings, is another imprecise exercise in present day medicine. Statistical definition of normal is the mean$\pm$ 2 Standard Deviation in a Gaussian distribution. This would automatically declare 5 per cent of the normal population as abnormal—the so-called false positives. This number (5%) goes up to 15—25% when we try to apply disease statistics to healthy people! This is very frightening when one takes the present hi-tech diagnostic gadgets into consideration. Let us look at the total body scanner that measures up to five hundred body parameters at a given time.

Well Man

When we check one hundred normal people using the total body scanner, therefore, two thousand five hundred abnormalities would be detected in those hundred normal people, even without their having any illness whatsoever. This would make us all abnormal in some sense or the other. **There will be no "well" human beings at all if one follows the modern medical evidence. A well man would be one who does not see any doctor. When he goes to see a doctor to get investigated he becomes a patient. Rarely ever does he have a chance to become well again.**

Reductionist Science

Medicine still follows reductionist science. We study organs through the study of the function of their cells. This is then projected on to the organ and finally we assume that the human body follows all our rules of deterministic predictability on the lines of Newtonian thinking. This has been the bane of medicine ever since modern medicine was accepted as science by the European Universities in the twelfth century. Although physics took the right route to unravel the mysteries of nature with the advent of quantum physics, modern medicine did not take notice. It is still mired in the time-honored Cartesian logic of reductionism. Modern science, including physics, has reached a stage where it needs to be rewritten with the discovery of human consciousness as the basis to try to understand nature. Everything is in the eye of the beholder. Almost all our studies so far have been flawed. Let us look at them in greater detail as we go along. Suffice it to say, at this stage, that we need to go back to the age old wisdom of holism followed both by the west before Rene Descartes, and by Indian and Chinese sciences for thousands of years. Deterministic predictability is a myth. The doctrine of probabilities, first enunciated by Blaise Pascal, a parish priest, when called to arbitrate in a game of dice, comes closer to truth even today.

Holistic Science

Human body works as a whole. The different organs do not function independently. They are all connected together and are under the influence of the most dominant rhythm of breathing. This concept is called "mode-locking" in physics. For example, the heart rate varies according to the phases of respiration—heart rate variability. The cardiac rhythm probably originates in the brain and not in the heart as was thought in the past. Newer specialties of neuro-cardiology and the like are coming up. Time evolution—what happens to a given man days, months, or years later—depends only on the total knowledge of that man initially. Modern medicine today is not in a position to assess a man completely as man is only thirty per cent phenotype (body features), another thirty per cent depends on his genes and the remaining forty per cent depends on the mind (consciousness). We are able to, may be, to asses a small fraction of the phenotype only at the present state of knowledge. In that background, doctors have been predicting the unpredictable future of mankind all through the history of modern medicine. This nullifies almost all of our statistical projections on to the population of our controlled studies for drug effectiveness or even the long-term outcome of elective prophylactic surgical procedures like coronary bypass etc. Controlled studies are further flawed because we are comparing a few body parameters of the two cohorts to match them while they have millions of other variables that we cannot assess at all with our present knowledge. No two individuals are alike, even twins have their variations!

Drug Studies

All our drug studies that we swear by have major errors. Firstly, at the drug discovery phase there are a couple of problems. A chemical molecule is discovered in the laboratory and then this is checked for its potency, toxicity, and other dynamic features usually using an animal model. There are now serious problems for animal studies all over the world. In an exhaustive study to be published in the European journal *Biogenic Amines* in May 2005, Jarrod Bailey, of the School of Population and Health Sciences at the University of Newcastle Upon Tyne in England has shown that animal-based drug tests could miss half of all birth defects. He feels that the next thalidomide could be just round the corner (*Good Medicine,* Spring 2005). The animal data is then extrapolated to man and preliminary studies are done on volunteers. If all these are uneventful, the final phase of drug development, the controlled study is mounted. We have looked at the problems besetting these studies. In addition, all the controlled studies are done for not longer than five years before the drug is let lose on the gullible public. Occasionally, the last step is even given a go before letting patients have the drug, with disastrous consequences. Many of the unforeseen side effects occur only after five years when the drug has been given to millions of people. Similar is the fate of surgical interventions and many other medical interventions.

Sexed-up Studies

Research funds drying up from independent sources, more and more studies are done with industry sponsorship. Most of them have strings attached. Positive reports have better chance of publication, the sponsors many times indulge in data dredging in addition, and occasionally companies get doctors to create diseases to sell drugs. It is a multibillion dollar business anyway and market forces influence research in this area very significantly. Academic medicine seems to be on sale these days with doctors and researchers being offered lavish gifts by the companies. Even the textbooks are written with drug company money! Final blow comes from researchers trying to confuse the doctors with complicated statistical methods when the data are not convenient to their mentors.

Evidence-burdened Medicine

For a conscientious doctor it is very difficult to practice medicine with the evidence produced. If he does not do that he would be liable to be sued for malpractice. If he follows every single datum pouring into the field at the Medline figures of seven per cent per month, I am sure, any practising doctor would be in a serious dilemma. One glaring example is the area of hypertension treatment. Whereas there are more than six guidelines in the world for doctors to follow, if all of them are computed together, the inclusion criteria add up to only 39% of patients. The majority of 61% do not have guidelines at all. Similarly, there are as many studies eulogizing coronary interventions as there are which show the former in very bad light.

In conclusion, one wonders as to how we have not taken note of all these glaring loopholes in the present system of medical science to rectify the same using better holistic methods of medical care. Modern medicine has become mandatory form emergency use anyway, but in the long term most of our interventions have been shown in very poor light. Another area of confusion is in understanding the words health care and medical care. The two are not synonymous. They are complementary. Health care needs basic amenities for the people and the quick-fix medical care interventions described above are for the minority that is ill and not fit for those who are well. The present effort is to use medical care methods for all, resulting in much misery and problems. Recently studies did show that when interventions come down death rate in the population falls down significantly. Time has come for right thinking doctors to wake up from their deep slumber to get out of their brainwashing by the industry to do most good to most people most of the time. A good doctor can never be dispensed with. He/she is then placebo for the human immune system to help heal the sick. May that tribe of placebo doctors increase!

Further reading

- Hegde BM. To do or not to do-Doctor's dilemma. *Kuwait Med J* 2001; 33(2): 107–110.
- Firth WJ. Chaos-Predicting the unpredictable. *BMJ* 1991; 303: 1565–1568.
- Editor. *Cecil's textbook of Medicine* 2002, 21st Edition. Page 1202.
- Hully S, Grady D, Bush T et al. Randomized trial of oestrogen plus progestin for secondary prevention of coronary heart disease in post-menopausal women. *JAMA* 1998; 280: 605–613

- McCormack J and Greenhalgh T. Seeing what you want to see in randomized controlled trials: versions and perversions of UKPDS data. *BMJ* 2000; 320: 1720–23.
- Krumholz HM. Cardiac procedures, outcomes, and accountability. *N Engl J Med* 1997; 336: 1522–23.
- Angell M. Is academic medicine for sale? *N Engl J Med* 2000; 342: 1516–8.
- Editorial. Drug Company influence on medical education in USA. *Lancet* 2000; 356: 781–83.
- Gribbin J. *In search of Schrodinger's cat.* 1991. Transworld Publishers, 61–63, Uxbridge Road, London W5 5 SA.
- Hegde BM, Shetty MA, and Shetty MR. *Hypertension-Assorted Topics.* Book. 1997. Bharathiya Vidya Bhavan, Bombay.
- Holmberg L, Bill-Axelson A, Helgesen F et al. A randomised trial comparing radical prostatectomy with watchful witting in early prostate cancer. *N Engl J Med* 2002; 347: 781–89.
- Andersson OK, Almgren T, Persson B et al. Survival in treated hypertension: follow up after two decades. *BMJ* 1998; 317: 167–171.

CHAPTER 30

Is Cancer a Disease?

The title does tickle, doesn't it? Does it make you think? If it did, my job will have been well done. There are maximum number of myths around this word **cancer**, the crab that really eats into the victim's body, and also his mind; the latter is the predominant disability of cancer, which needs **care and not cure.** Not a day passes without the news about miracles in cancer cures and unwanted premature deaths. It is the connection between death and disease that makes cancer that much more frightening. Man is ultimately afraid of dying. The medical fraternity keeps feeding society with all the wrong notions that diseases cause death. On the contrary, death is the only certainty in life, which has very little to do with disease. Diseases do cause disability, pain, and undue suffering. It should be the endeavour of the medical establishment to "cure rarely, comfort mostly, but to console always."

The basic truth about cancer seems to be far removed from all these myths. Cancer, in fact, is not a disease. It is a process of ageing—some of us age slowly, yet others age faster. I am talking of cell ageing and not of morphologic ageing. That explains cancers occurring even in small children. Depending on the rate of growth of a cancer, it could either outlive the victim or precede him. When the cancer starts to grow inside the human body there is always an attempt by the body's immune system to suppress it, or to overcome it. If, in the bargain, the immune system wins, the cancer dies prematurely. The unusually high incidence of cancers in those patients with AIDS clearly proves the point.

Biological cancer is a normal body cell, which has outlived its appointed time of death. Every cell in the human body, of which there are whopping one hundred thousand billion in all, have their life span cut out for them. They have to die a natural death, apoptosis (falling of a brown leaf, in Greek). A special gene, the suicide gene, which sends the message to every cell, when its time is up, governs this process. With such large number of cells belonging to so many varieties of organs and tissues, one shudders to think as to how this goes on in the majority of us without a hitch! If, for any reason, the suicide gene either fails to send the signal, or the messenger enzymes do not do their job well, the target cell might not receive the message at all. That cell could outlive its life span, but cannot divide any further, since there is an upper limit for cell replication in every situation (Hayflick's law). The cell that escapes death at the right time **mutates** to change its DNA, called the rogue DNA. *The latter is the beginning of a potential future cancer, if it chooses to do so.*

It is, therefore, possible that every human being has some potential cancer or the other at all times. It is only an accident that one such could really become a clinical cancer. Ottoson in Sweden did minute postmortem study of two hundred and fifty consecutive deaths due to suicide, where he found the presence of a biological cancer in every one of them. Depression is the cause of suicide. Depression is now known to be associated with cancer, heart attacks, and many other major illnesses.

Clinical cancer is that stage where the rogue DNA of the cell replicates thousands of times to produce a mass of cells that could be felt as a lump (tumour) by the doctor. Even this stage of clinical cancer could be dormant for years on end, depending on the site of the lump. When that chooses to grow rapidly and/or to grow at distant sites in addition, causing local pressure symptoms, depending on the site and the function of the organ, the victim feels the symptoms due to the growth; this stage is called **symptomatic cancer**. Even then it could, at times, remain dormant for years on end. At the other end of the spectrum is the tumour that could grow very fast, and produce symptoms that are disabling in a very short span of time.

What is Early Cancer?

This is the greatest myth of the century. There is no way one could detect cancer at its biological stage. Even if we could do that hypothetically, there is no way we could gauge if it is going to be a clinical cancer or not. Even at the stage of clinical cancer we have no means of saying which cancer grows and at what pace. It is near nigh impossible, by the available means, to say what would be the outcome of the cancer. Even the cytological diagnosis of cancer is only a guess; as cancer cells are, after all, normal cells with some difference. The cytological diagnosis, at times, is very tricky and difficult. Most of the time a diagnosis is a false positive one for defensive purposes. **Scientifically there is nothing called early cancer from the prognostic point of view.** Thomas Lewis, the former President of the world famous Sloane Kettering Cancer Institute in New York, wrote in his famous book *The Lives of a Cell* that:

"Illness and death still exist and cannot be hidden. We are still beset by plain diseases, and we do not control them; they are loose on their own, afflicting as unpredictably and haphazardly. We are only able to deal with them when they make their appearance (it is better to conserve our meagre resources just for that!)...Majority of cancers can neither be prevented nor cured. We do not become sick because of failure of vigilance, diseases do not happen just because we are not preserving health."

There is nothing called early cancer; any cancer even if it is discovered "very early" could be decades old biologically and could have had the seedlings in distant organs already. The concept of early cancer is a very good business for the screening industry though, which thrives on that myth. Teleologically, one needs to intervene only when the so-called cancer starts to produce symptoms. We have very good methods of palliation, *but no cure whatsoever for cancer as of now in 2005*. No one, not even the best oncologist, could predict with certainty, as to the future course of the disease. They have, of course, been predicting the unpredictable, again a good business proposition!

Role of Cancer Screening

This is another one of those myths sustained by intense propaganda in the medical world. Audit of allmost all the properly conducted screening studies has given equivocal results. This is very obvious in the field of gynaecological cancers. Judged by the enormity of the problem this propaganda is well worth the effort and the money spent on it. In one year in the USA alone, 600,000 hysterectomies (uterus removals) were done for preventing cancers, based on the screening data. The story of mammograms has been still more interesting. Some governments have, at last, put a moratorium on screening young ladies. There are a couple of unconfirmed reports that wonder if mammograms could even stimulate a biologic cancer to grow faster! Although the incidence of breast cancer is very high in elderly ladies, there is very little done in that age group.

There are stray reports that early detection of cancers in their presymptomatic stage might send the wrong signal of a death sentence to the harassed patient that makes the cancer grow faster, to produce its deleterious effects on the organ concerned. The resultant disability might even kill the victim faster. It is a well-known fact that fear could kill! Cancer could be predicted in the herd, but not in the individual. The incidence of herd cancer has not changed a wee bit over the last few decades although individual cancer incidences have shown changes. For example, the Japanese have very low incidence of stomach cancers but they compensate by very high incidence of many other cancers, compared to the Americans. The overall incidence has not changed though the numbers are higher, obviously because there are more people in the world now compared to the past!

Are Cancers Hereditary?

Herd cancers are hereditary. In individuals, there is no unequivocal proof that cancers are hereditary. Environment and genes work together in any disease.

What about Cancer Treatment?

It is another one of those medical myths. Small is as good as large would be a good surgical dictum in cancer surgery. The heroic surgery, with the poor patient in the hero's role, are many times counterproductive. Scientific studies have amply proved that lumpectomy, or local surgery to clear the pressure symptoms, are as good as the most radical extensive mutilating surgeries. The final outcome did not appreciably differ in such heroic patients. Repeated surgeries are another thing altogether. This was practised even in the distant past. Sigmund Freud had thirty-three operations over a period of sixteen years for his oral cancer. He did not die, though!

Chemotherapy and radiation are again done for the overkill. Both these could kill normal cells as well as cancer cells. In fact, they kill fast growing cells more effectively, resulting in hair loss, oral mucus membrane loss, loss of testicular function, and the like. There is now a growing feeling that chemotherapy and radiation also should be done just about enough for good palliation, and symptom relief, rather than for *radical cure.* The latter is a pure myth in cancer. One of world's leading oncologists, Sir David Wetherall, Regius Professor of Medicine at the Oxford University, wrote in his recent book *The Science of Medicine and its Quiet Art* (Oxford Publications, 1997) thus:

"The way we burn our cancer patients with powerful drugs and radiation reminds one of the branding done routinely for diseases by our forefathers. Our future generation will not forgive us for this blunder."

Having said all this, I am aware of the anger and wrath I shall incur from my friends and colleagues. I used to get upset about it when I was young, but I have grown to ignore that now. I was reading in the recent issue of the *British Medical Journal* about the lamentations of its brilliant editor, Richard Smith, about the abuses heaped on him week after week, when his journal reaches the readers: "The earlier you are fired the better for the nation", "You should end up as a street sweeper after being fired from the editorship of the BMJ" etc. I am not alone in this world in my travails. There is good company. Richard Smith is a very fine man and an excellent scientist, in addition, he has been considered one of the ablest editors of that prestigious journal, which has undergone sea of change after Richard took up the challenge as its editor! After 25 years as the editor, Richard now has a six figure salary job with an American conglomerate! Good luck Richard!

If what I have written gives courage to the hapless victims of cancer, and makes my colleagues to start thinking, my efforts will have been amply rewarded. Cancer need not kill always—with or without treatment. Fear kills faster! Cancer might even keep one alive and kicking for as long as thirty to forty years. If one takes its biological state into consideration, it could be even fifty to sixty years. Many cancers, especially of the prostate gland, have outlived their owners! Happiness of the mind is known to kill cancers or suppress their growth, while depression is known to stimulate biologically quiescent cancers to grow very rapidly and wildly.

Prasanna aatham indriya manaha Swastha Ithyabhideeyathe.
(Happiness keeps you healthy!)

Never try to live for ever, you will certainly not succeed,

—Bernard Shaw in *Doctor's Dilemma*

Further Reading

- Thomas Lewis. *Lives of a Cell.* 1987. Harper Collins.
- Bailar JC and Gornik HL. Cancer Undefeated. *New England Journal of Medicine* 1997;336:1569–1574

CHAPTER 31

Interventional Cardiology

> **Great minds discuss ideas,**
> **Average minds discuss events,**
> **Small minds discuss people.**
>
> —*Anon*

Our education being replicative, it does not allow us to think about our learning material. If one has to learn from one's own experience, he should be able to do a bit of introspection. We seem to believe everything that we read for our examinations, as gospel truth. Rarely do we develop the capacity to question the published knowledge. David Eddy, a former associate professor of cardiovascular surgery at the Stanford University, came to the interesting conclusion, after extensive study of the medical literature, that **"eighty five per cent of what doctors do is based on soft data; only fifteen per cent is based on hard unequivocal data."** This applies to textbooks as well.

New Statesman once quoted a high school student who said:

> **Sciences are learning facts from a book**
> **and not thinking for yourself,**
> **I wanted to express my own ideas and then think for myself!**

Why do we do what we do, then? Many wise teachers have answered this million-dollar question and, I only have, herein, attempted to quote a few of them. I shall not impose my ideas on the reader at this point in time, but let the reader draw his/her own conclusions. Please remember that medical muddling is a good business. Professor Krumholz, cardiologist at the Yale, wrote in an editorial in the *New England Journal of Medicine,* regarding an audit of post-infarction revascularization, *"In a fee-for-service system, cardiac procedures generated billions of dollars in revenues each year. A high volume of procedures brought prestige and financial rewards for hospitals, physicians, and the vendors of medical equipment."* One could easily grasp the motive behind these procedures in cardiology. If that were so in the USA, what of our corporate hospitals elsewhere? There is always the profit motive in these ventures that make the employee to **perform or perish.** Most of us are skilled labour in this new hospital industry! The initial investments in costly cardiac equipment would, perforce, demand higher returns to pay both the staff and the banks! Young interventionists are, therefore, egged on to do more and more.

This situation brings to mind the saying of Mark Twain:

For a man with a hammer in the hand and wanting to use it, everything here looks like a nail needing hammering.

The above adage is shown to be true in interventional cardiology, by two landmark papers. The first one is by the Harvard group, led by Nobel Laureate Bernard Lown, in the *JAMA*. The study showed that only three percent of the 200 patients referred to their centre for CABG by local cardiologists, scientifically needed the procedure. The rest were followed up for fifteen long years without any adverse effects. The authors advocated *"stricter control at the level of an angiogram in the diagnosis of coronary disease. Angiogram is indicated only as a prerequisite for plumbing, and should only be done after the decision to revascularise is made on the patient's clinical condition. Done earlier, this might frighten the patient and relatives into agreeing for the procedure unnecessarily."*

Next is the advice by one of the leading professors of cardiac surgery in England, Tom Treasure, who in his paper in *The Lancet,* strongly pleaded for reducing cardiac angiography set ups in the UK to avoid their overuse. Professor Hampton, of the Nottingham University, found in one of his studies that in his area more than 47% of the angiograms were inappropriately done. Dr Tu and colleagues in Yale found, in a comparative study of Philadelphia in the US and Ontario, in Canada, that the intervention ratio, in the immediate post-infarction period in these two identical populations was 7.8:1. Surprisingly, at the end of the year there were almost equal numbers of those patients alive in both the places!

Another audit of sixty thousand bypass surgeries done in the US showed that only 14 per cent did get survival benefit, ranging from three months to four and a half years. A good 84% did not get any extra life.

One would be surprised that there are quite a few small and medium studies, published even in good journals, which extol the virtues of bypass and angioplasty, although no large controlled study has ever shown that. How do the smaller studies show good results? If one wants to get any clue to this disparity, one has to *overstand the* subject and not just *understand* it, as we do. Many of these studies are funded by vested interests. A recent meta-analysis showed how these studies could be engineered. In a mile stone paper in the April 1999 issue of the *JAMA*, Drs. Campbell and colleagues at the Harvard, showed how research related gifts is a common and important form of research support. The title of the paper makes interesting reading: *"Looking a gift horse in the mouth-corporate gifts supporting Life Science Research!"*

Even in other areas of drug intervention, the story is no different. Cardiogenic shock is the leading cause of death among people admitted with myocardial infarction, and it remains the same even today as it was 35 years ago. Reperfusion treatments including thrombolysis seem to have made no impact on the incidence of cardiogenic shock, which occurs in about 5–15% of patients with heart attack. Very aggressive reperfusion may have helped to improve short-term survival only.

Whereas ACE inhibitors did help patients after a heart attack associated with clinical evidence of heart failure in the *AIRE study*, the same did not hold well in all patients given ACE inhibitors de novo routinely. Nature must have been trying to help the ventricle after a heart attack by *remodeling*. The latter is assisted by the ACE system. Only when Nature fails and the victim suffers the ill effects by way of heart failure, do ACE inhibitors help a great deal. Could ACE inhibitors alter the remodeling process? Even in a study of diabetics on insulin therapy, symptomatic patients alone got benefit in their quality of life. The asymptomatic ones did not get any benefit!

In the MRC study of mild–moderate hypertension, it was shown that to save one patient from stroke in the long run nearly 850 patients needed unnecessary treatment for years on end. Even the recent *HOT* study gave us a warning! While the vigorously treated group did have its BP recording brought down to the ideal range, death rate did go up in that group; an instance of the **euboxic philosophy** of modern western medicine, viz.: the case-sheet of the patient must have all the parameters within the normal range. It matters very little if the patient dies in the bargain, as long as all the boxes in the case sheet are correctly marked—euboxic death.

We could, instead, try and keep a patient alive, with the boxes still slightly skewed, a stage I would like to call as dysboxic *life.* Long-term follow up of two cohorts of Finnish men, one vigorously intervened and the other left to tend for itself as and when needed, showed that the intervened group had much higher cardiovascular and total death compared to the usual care group! Most of the anti-arrhythmic drugs did, at the end of the day, result in higher deaths in the treated group compared to the controls in the *CAST* study.

Epidemics of vascular diseases are being predicted daily to scare the public and get them to the screening centres in large numbers. Stehaben's extensive studies did not show any real increase in the incidence of vascular diseases in the last one hundred years. It is now known that routine screening, in certain situations, might even endanger the patients' lives, if one cares to read the editorial *Screening could be dangerous to your health* in the *BMJ (1997)! Do epidemiologists cause epidemics?* is an editorial in the *Lancet (1993)*, giving timely warning to our interventionists. Unfortunately, screening healthy populations makes very good business sense. While there could be a few million sick at a given point in time, there would be billions who could be detected to have occult pathologies of dubious future significance, when routinely screened. Many might even get worse after labeling! The industry would, of course, opt for the latter. Executive check-ups are a very good fishing net to have bigger catches.

Diagnostic tests are another area where we overdo testing in a big way. While good clinical sense could get most accurate diagnoses in the majority, routine tests like stress test and echocardiograms could throw up false positives in a big way. Rudimentary knowledge of statistics would tell us that the disease-based statistics applied to the vast healthy populations should, per force, bring about large numbers of false positives.

Whereas the specificity and sensitivity of the stress test depends, to a great extent, on the prevalence of the coronary disease in the population, we predict the unpredictable by looking at the ST-T changes in the electrocardiogram, even without having any clue about the prevalence of the disease in our population! Cardiac neurosis has gone up exponentially in recent years after these tests were introduced, more so because these tests are done and interpreted, in many cases, by centers with inadequate experience.

It is our bounden duty to do our best for the suffering humanity as doctors, but when it comes to professing to help the apparently healthy, through the screening procedures in society, we are on a very wet wicket, indeed.

Come to think of it, one of the many meanings of the word intervene, is **to go in between with malice!** My only fond hope is that our divine interventionists do not aim at that.

That said, I must hasten to add that many of the interventions, like bypass surgery, are a real boon to the badly suffering patients with coronary disease. Where angina is intractable, and/or the left ventricular function is really depressed, bypass surgery gives great relief to the victim, making life worth living. We should not deify ourselves by saying that these interventions, which are purely palliative, are going to keep man alive here forever and would avoid sudden death etc. Let me remind the reader of the warning given by Bernard Shaw in his book *Doctor's Dilemma* saying: "do not try to live for ever, you will certainly not succeed." In fact, the incidence of sudden death is not altered by bypass surgery. The prolongation of life is only a mirage. Symptom relief and better quality of life are certainly the blessings.

In conclusion, I have presented here data from the same *"authentic"* sources that one gets all other data about the other side of the coin in modern medicine. *I am not trying to say that we should be therapeutic nihilists.* **My only plea is that we, as a profession, should let the gullible public know the real truth, to let them be equal partners in their own management.** The **"paternalistic"** attitude in medicine is not good; which has taken medicine to the market place. Market forces have made medicine prohibitively expensive. In addition, market forces equate us with the other traders, exposing us to the ravages of consumerism. "Never make money in the sick room" was one of the Hippocratic aphorisms.

Dr Glenn JR Whitman, chief surgeon at the University of Maryland Medical Centre, explains that the complications of bypass surgery are multiplied by the time taken on the bypass machine. He goes on to say: "Having your blood pass through a plastic tube during surgery is not good for you. God didn't make our blood go through a pump outside of us."

I would request you to contemplate on what I have written and then draw your own conclusions. **You could go back and do what you want to do.** Science, in every sphere, is dying slowly because of specialization. New science of fractals and chaos looks at the dynamic human being as a whole, and as a part of this macrocosm. That is the future of science, including our medical science. In this era of exciting scopes and interventions we should never lose sight of the art of medicine.

"Art" is defined best by Henry David Thoreau as ***"that which makes the man's day."*** The art of medicine is that which makes the patients' day. The intervention might be divine; but its aim should be to make the patient feel better at the end of the day! Medicine revolves round ***anxiety***— patient anxiety of disability and death, and the doctor anxiety of doing more and more. Doctors, including interventionists, should try and allay these anxieties and not add to it. Long live medicine which aims to ***"cure rarely, comfort mostly, but console always." Let us try to do most good to most people most of the time.*** The old meaning of science that "Science is what scientists do", originally written in Dutch as "Wotenchap is wat wotenchoppers doen," has been proved wrong by the new meaning of science, what with its Sanskrit root "*skei*", meaning to "***cut into***" everything you observe!

> **We do not see things as they are,**
> **We see them as we are.**
>
> —Nin Anais

Further Reading

- Krumholz HM. Cardiac Procedures, outcomes, and accountability. *N Engl J Med* 1997; 336; 1522–23.
- Graboys TB, Biegelson B, Lampwert S, Blatt CM, & Lown B. Second Opinion trial of Coronary angiography. *JAMA* 1992; 268: 2537–2540.
- Treasure T. US doubts about angiography. *Lancet* 1993; 341: 154.

- Gray D, Hampton JR, Bernstein S et al. Audit of coronary arteriography and bypass. *Lancet* 1990; 335; 1317–1320.
- Tu JV, Pashos CL, Naylor DC et al. Use of cardiac procedures and their outcome in elderly patients in US and Canada. *N Engl J Med* 1997; 336:1500–1505.
- Hux JE, Naylor DC. In the eye of the beholder. *Arch Intern Med* 1995; 155: 2277–2280.
- Loop FD. Coronary artery surgery: the end of the beginning. *Eur J Cardiothorac Surg*. 1998; 14(6): 554–571.
- Campbell EG, Louis KS, Blumenthal D. Looking a gift horse in the mouth. *JAMA* 1999; 279: 995–999.
- Goldberg RJ, Samad NA, Yarzebski J, et al. Temporal trends in Cardiogenic shock complicating AMI. *N Engl J Med* 1999; 340: 1162–1168.
- Ball SG, Hall SA, Macintosh AF et al. Effect of ramipril and morbidity of survivors of AMI with clinical evidence of clinical heart failure. *Lancet* 1993; 342: 821–828.

- Kober L, Torp Pederson C, Carlsen JE et al. Clinical trial of ACE inhibitor-trandelopril in LV dysfunction after AMI. *N Engl J Med* 1995; 333: 1670–1676.
- Goddijn PPM, Bilo HJG, Feskens EJM et al. Longitudinal study of glycaemic control. *Diabet Med* 1999; 16: 23–30.
- MRC Study Group. Treatment of mild-moderate hypertension-Principal results. *BMJ* 1985; 291: 97–104.
- Chalmers J: Hot Study: brilliant concept, but a qualified success. *J Hypertens.* 1998; 16(10):1403–1405.
- Davidoff F. *Who has seen a blood sugar?* Book. 1998. American College of Physicians.
- Nacarelli GV, Wolbrette DL, Dell Orfano JT, et al. CAST to AVID and beyond. *J Cardiovasc Electrophysiol.* 1998; 9(8): 864–91.
- Stehabens WJ. An appraisal of the epidemic rise of coronary artery disease and its decline. *Lancet* 1987;I: 606–611.
- Stewart-Brown S, Farmer A. Screening could seriously damage your health. *BMJ* 1997; 314: 533.
- Editorial. Do epidemiologists cause epidemics? *Lancet* 1993; 341: 993–994
- Redwood DR, Borer JS, Epstein SE. Whither ST segment during exercise? *Circulation* 1976; 54:703-706.
- Hegde BM. The unrest cure. *J Assoc Physi India.* 1997; 47: 730–731.
- Richard O'Mara. Heart Surgery: Does off-pump beat the pump. *Indian Express*, March 13th 1999.
- Hegde BM. Chaos- a new concept in science. *J Assoc Physi India* 1996; 44: 167–68.
- Hegde BM. The science of medicine. Ibid. 1998; 46: 896–97.
- Pickering WG. Does medical treatment mean patient benefit? *Lancet* 1996;347: 379–80.

CHAPTER 32

Is Artificial Heart a Reality?

British Medical Journal of the 12th August 2000 carries the exciting news item that the first artificial heart had been transplanted into a patient in terminal heart failure very successfully. The operation was performed in Jerusalem by an Israeli surgeon. The operation lasted for twelve long hours and the patient is said to have recovered after the operation to the satisfaction of all concerned. Of course, as usual, the patient did die after three and half days of the operation. "The patient died of multi-organ failure, but his implanted artificial heart was found to be functioning well right up to the time of his death!" said the hospital spokeswoman.

Here is good news and bad news, both together. Good news is that the device, the price of which is not mentioned, has been tested to be working in a human being for the first time. The bad news is that the patient died so soon after the surgery. One could blame so many factors for the death. In fact, the surgeon who operated went on record to say that the patient "would have lived for a few hours only if the operation was not performed. His condition was such that he had one foot in his grave already." How did this divine doctor come to know the exact life span of this poor patient is anybody's guess. I am not aware of any medical scientific method of accurately predicting somebody's death.

This new device is called **Heart Mate II** and is manufactured by a company in Pittsburgh, Pennsylvania, Thermo Cardiosystems. The company which originally devised the artificial heart was the Developing Artificial Organs Centre in Pittsburgh. It is a small device weighing only 350 gm, powered by a lithium battery. This device had been tried in animals earlier and it did show good working for long periods of time. Being a small device it does not replace the heart. It is in fact only a left ventricular assist device. It could be implanted in the abdomen to pump oxygenated blood through the left ventricle to all parts of the body. The other chambers of the heart work in tandem with the device. Since most heart failures basically are left ventricular failures this device could work like an artificial heart. Like the implanted pacemaker it could have life long power supply systems attached to it if it functions well inside the human body.

The unanswered question, however, is the reason why this device was not tried first in the USA? Dr Jacob Lavee, the chief of cardiovascular surgery at the Sheba Hospital in Tel Aviv, claims that his selection as the world's first surgeon to have done this feat is because of his training in Pittsburgh for a year in 1989–90, although there were many aspirants in Europe who wanted to be the first. I am sure Indian surgeons would have tried their best if they had a chance to be the first in the field.

Reporters asked surgeon Lavee as to why the US surgeons were shying away. His answer has all the hidden agenda in such situations: "**The Food and Drug Administration in the US does not permit its use there unless they are shown that it works in 30–50 human patients elsewhere.**"

It is not out of place here to remind one of the first ever heart transplant in humans by Christian Bernard in South Africa. Dr Bernard's former mentor, Norman Shumway, at the Stanford University, was the one who perfected the original technique. Now that Bernard does not have much respect for his teacher, he does not admit that he climbed to fame riding piggyback on Norman. He claimed in one of his recent interviews with Dimbleby of the BBC that the original idea was that of the father of British cardiac surgery, Sir Russell Brock. Be that as it may, the truth still is that the first operation was done neither in the US nor the UK, but in far off South Africa; that too the donor heart came from a black man at the height of the Apartheid regime!

The crux of the matter is that all these new devices are being tested to see if they work in humans in countries other than the advanced West. These particular operators have been silent on the miserable state in which the recipient lived for the next four days in the intensive therapy unit. He must have been kept alive with the technology in a vegetative state to claim the success of the procedure. Even if one were to believe the story of the surgeons at the Sheba Hospital that the patient would have otherwise lived for a few hours but died four days later instead the fact remains that it did not do any good anyway! Operation successful but patient died is the usual story.

Terminal heart failure is a state in which many other organs are also badly compromised in their functioning capacity. With the earliest sign of heart failure, when the patient is still asymptomatic, there are many changes in the vital organs and other organ functions to keep the patient going on for a long time. If this compensatory phase gets upset and the person starts to get symptoms, the vital organs suffer all the more. By the time the patient reaches the terminal stage of failure, where such expensive devices are indicated, many organs that keep the man alive are as bad, if not worse, than the heart. No organ in the human body works in isolation to be easily replaced by a new organ or a device to get the owner back to normalcy. This statement applies to the heart all the more, as it is the pump that gives the life-sustaining oxygen to every cell in the human body. The longer does the heart suffer in the state of failure greater will be the damage to all other organs.

That is the main reason why heart transplants and artificial devices in that situation would not be as useful as in kidney transplant for that matter. The latter could be transplanted to do its limited function and post-transplant survival there is much better. All the sophisticated technologies could only palliate and never cure the condition. The very concept of quick fixes like the one described above defeat the very purpose of medicine. The highest technology is that which eradicates a disease. More work needs to be done to see why people get heart failure in the first place and to find out ways and means of preventing heart failure, if possible.

Another lesson that we learn from the present tragedy is that human being should be viewed as whole and not in bits and pieces. It is unfortunate that we still believe Rene Descartes when he wrote in the seventeenth century that he believes that since the body is divisible and the mind is indivisible, the mind and body are separate. This mind–body dualism and the consequent reductionist science have been our biggest bane in medical science. The mother of all medical wisdoms, Ayurveda, looks at the human body as a whole and as a part of this macrocosm. More research in that area using the modern technological touchstone could solve more problems for mankind than the entire hi-tech put together. Said Karl Popper, a great thinker: "Knowledge advances not by **repeating** known facts but by **refuting** false dogmas."

Writing in his book, *Lives of a Cell,* Thomas Lewis classifies technology as high, medium and low. He concludes by saying that the only one low-tech method that has eradicated the only disease, small pox, is vaccination. This originally from the ancient Indian system of vaccination followed for "times out of mind" in that country. It was TZ Hollwell, FRCP(London), FRS, that came to India in the 18th Century to study Indian vaccination system and stayed on for 20 years and wrote about its efficacy to the President of the Royal College of Physicians of London in the year 1747. That gave credibility to the anecdotal experience of Edward Jenner. After 1747 incident only, vaccination became accepted as scientific method to prevent small pox.

FURTHER READING

- Hegde BM. Vaccination in India. *J Assoc Physicians India.* 1998; 47: 472–473.

CHAPTER 33

Life Expectancy Versus Health Expectancy

Modern hi-tech medicine claims that it has increased human **life expectancy.** In fact, life expectancy started increasing with better food supply, control of communicable diseases, and better education of the masses making them live a healthier life style. In developing poor countries life expectancy could have a quantum jump if only **infant mortality comes down.** Life expectancy is a statistical term, which does not mean that **human life span** has increased in this century due to all the hi-tech stuff that we are trying to sell to the gullible public! On the contrary, life span has, if anything, come down from the usual 120–140 years that some of the aboriginal races in certain pockets of the world still enjoy. It is now estimated that the average American life expectancy cannot go beyond 89 years even in the next millennium.

What is life expectancy?

If a mother gives birth to ten children and if eight of them die around birth, as used to happen in many parts of the poor nations, even if the other two children live up to 100 years, the life expectancy of another child being born to any mother in similar settings would be **only twenty years** (100 multiplied by 2 and divided by 10). This could change dramatically if instead of eight children dying around birth, only four die and the rest live for 100 years, the life expectancy in that setting would jump to 60 years! Now one could understand the meaning of the word life expectancy. The change in life expectancy, therefore, has very little to do with the so-called hi-tech curative medicine.

What is Life Span?

The maximum number of years any species (Homo sapiens) could live is called **life span.** This is fixed, as early as the day one is made in the mother's womb, in the genetic material. This cannot and would not change with even the highest technological efforts. Hayflick's rule gives each cell its maximum capacity to reproduce and apoptosis tells the cells when to die (in certain cells like the heart muscle cell there is no apoptosis under normal circumstances). Recent efforts to increase the life span by genetic engineering also have come to naught, as senescence could not be halted in those modified cells. It is no use having a 150-year-old very senile vegetable in society! The latter would be a burden on society, any way. Life span has remained the same since the dawn of the human race.

What is Health Expectancy?

This is a neologism introduced by me. It is the time interval between birth and the end of healthy life—before the onset of any major incapacitating illness. Man is **healthy only when he is creative in society. Absence of physical illness is not the complete definition of health. In fact, many people with physical diseases are more creative, and consequently healthier, than their counterparts in society without any physical disease, but having no enthusiasm.** Thus defined, health becomes a very useful commodity in society. In fact, healthy people in society could even make society more tranquil. Crime of every kind, from petty theft to murder and terrorism are all signs of disease (dis-ease)—not of the body but of the mind. Mental illnesses are not only depression and schizophrenia. Aberrant behaviour patterns should also fall into that category.

Now let us critically examine if the present day scientific hi-tech methods have increased health expectancy in society. The most advanced country in the world, United States of America, probably is the unhealthiest country in the world with the **lowest health expectancy, despite the fact that Americans have a very healthy life style among the white races!** Health screening surveys there have shown, in larger cities like New York, that every other man has either high blood pressure, heart disease or diabetes. There is hardly anyone who has not seen a doctor for a major illness or has had some surgical procedure done on him or is taking some kind of a medicine or another at any given time. Crime is on the increase, novel methods are being discovered now and then. Even high school students resort to shooting their own classmates in school!

Time has come for us to ponder over this tragedy very seriously. Professor Eiesenburg, an American professor of medicine, recently wrote to say that a **truly well man is not available in America.** If all the available screening tests are used on every American all of them will have some sort of an abnormality or another, requiring intervention. In an interesting article, *The Last Well Man,* the author, an American doctor, laments on the present state of the art in this field. Our aim should be see that the majority of people in society have at least half their lifetime free of disease. The next millennium should aim at having the population's health expectancy come up to, at least, fifty years.

What are the Prerequisites for Attaining Decent Health Expectancy?

Clean water, adequate food supply, care of the pregnant woman, adequate pacing of pregnancy, universal literacy so that every one has access to information, avoiding tobacco and alcohol, avoiding dependence on others for any reason including religion, avoiding unhealthy competition in life which begets hostility, hard physical work or regular exercise for all, proper immunization methods in childhood, trying to live in a clean atmosphere without excess pollution, controlling the world population by reassuring the poor man that his children need not die prematurely in the new set up rather than selling contraceptive methods to him, empowering the poor man economically by narrowing the gulf between the haves and the have-nots in society and bringing up children, especially our adolescents, correctly should go a long way in achieving the health expectancy for the population of, at least, 50 years.

To cap it, we have to make man more tranquil by the ancient Indian methods of meditation and breathing techniques; the latter go a long way in postponing the onset of illness thereby increasing health expectancy. Prevention is better than cure may not be true always, but changing the mode of living of people is definitely cheaper than both the former. I hope we canalize our efforts in this direction rather than continuing the rat race of more and more technology for fire fighting (curative methods). The fire fighting hose seems to be perpetually short of its target!

Trying to change the mode of living of society is much cheaper in the long run and more effective than screening large populations for diseases and then trying to set them right. There is no guarantee that the change in the initial state of the organism (man) due to drug treatment or surgical intervention of the apparently healthy population is going to do good in the long run. The human body does not follow the linear mathematical rules! To give a concrete example: if one brings down the mildly elevated blood pressure in an apparently healthy man that in itself might not do any good; on the contrary, it may do more harm due to the side effects of long term drugging. Whereas trying to change his mode of living might bring the pressure down by the natural means for the long term good of the victim. Similar is the story with diabetes or even cancer.

Screening large populations is prohibitively expensive and only increases anxiety in society resulting in large-scale sick absenteeism. In a well-researched editorial in *The Lancet* the authors make out a good case against screening. The heading is very interesting to read: *Do Epidemiologists cause Epidemics?* **I think they do!** At the same wavelength is an editorial in *the British Medical Journal* entitled *Screening Could Seriously Damage Your Health.* I must congratulate the authors for their courage! They could not be more correct.

Why do we, then, Advocate Routine Screening of Healthy People?

I strongly feel, I may be wrong though, that routine screening is how the medi-business thrives. If the medical establishment were to tell the public the truth, the whole truth and nothing but the truth, then we should be content with treating the sick population only. There may be only a few million clients for the curative business at any given time. If on the other hand, we target the whole population there is a huge stock of six billion to draw from. The latter makes a lot of business sense. Logically the latter is better business. The multibillion-dollar drug industry, equipment manufacturing industry, and also the corporate hospital industry should thrive on this business, and it makes sense that they target a larger clientele.

Well meaning NGOs and the governments of poorer countries should read the writing on the wall that hi-tech top heavy modern medical interventions are not a panacea for man's ills but are a good quick fix for mending damaged organs. The long-term outcomes are anybody's guess. Doctors have been predicting the unpredictable! Let us put our heads together to see how best we could change the mode of living of man in the present world of cut throat competition.

Further Reading

- Editorial. Drug Company influence on medical education in USA. *Lancet* 2000; 356: 781–83.
- Stewart-Brown S, Farmer A. Screening could seriously damage your health. *BMJ* 1997; 314: 533.
- Editorial. Do epidemiologists cause epidemics? *Lancet* 1993; 341: 993–994

CHAPTER 34

Mitral Valve Prolapse Syndrome

The name is very familiar now but was not known before the late sixties and early seventies. With the advent of echocardiography newer diseases came to light! I still remember the days when we were playing with a simple mid-line echo machine used in neurology delineating the mid-line shift in the brain. We tried that on the heart and had to struggle for a long time to get at the anterior mitral leaflet. My paper on echocardiography in the Karnataka Medical Journal was possibly the first one in India. I have not been able to get any earlier reports so far. I had made a reference to this new syndrome in that paper and had stressed the need for caution in the diagnosis, since the technique of echocardiography had to be perfect to get the correct diagnosis. Even if the echo did show any change in the configuration of the mitral valve, that, by itself, does not make it a serious disease.

In a beautiful editorial in *The Lancet*, it was shown how epidemics of diseases could be caused by epidemiologists themselves. Labeling gives rise to awareness and the latter in turn results in overdiagnosis! The same holds good for vascular diseases like coronary artery disease these days. The new labels increase anxiety in the population. While our whole effort in medicine should aim at reducing anxiety, here is an effort to increase anxiety. Thousands of young men and mostly women have been frightened out of their wits by the new breed of cardiologists with their newly acquired echo machines. The more the merrier and newer the better is the slogan in this field now.

I am reminded of a personal anecdote. I was reviewing a middle aged woman in the outpatient cardiac clinic at the Middlesex Hospital, London in 1974. **This lady was seen as a school girl thirty years earlier by a great cardiologist, Even Bedford, in the same clinic.** The referral letter from the GP said: "I hear a peculiar sound at the apex. Please clarify if this is due to cardiac disease?" The wise old man, Evan Bedford, had written: "I do not think that this short mid-systolic murmur with a click is due to any cardiac pathology. You could reassure her on that count. However, to be on the safer side she could be reviewed here once in five years." The letter was still there in the file! I echocardiogrammed her that day and found mitral valve billowing. It was then called Billowing Mitral Leaflet Syndrome (BMLS) by Prof Barlow of South Africa. He, along with his able assistant Wendy Pocock, had contributed a lot to clear this mystery.

The middle aged lady was in the pink of her health and had two children by the time I reviewed her. Of course, I had to reassure her again. The wisdom of the wise old man struck me then. Since then lot of water has flowed under the bridge and people have made mountains out of mole hills of this minor alteration in the size of the chordae tendinae. How I wish we had appreciated Nature's ways better! People are told these days that any one with this kind of a change is in for serious problems in life like sudden death, infective endocarditis, mitral leaks with attendant consequences and so on and so forth. I do not think any one has given as much as a small thought to the anxiety and torture that are induced in the poor victims of our technological attacks on them. It may not be a bad idea for cardiologists to get into such **unfortunate people's shoes and think of their own lives with that kind of a death warrant given to them by their doctors.**

Now comes some relief for those poor victims. A large prospective and long term follow up study from the USA in the recent *New England Journal of Medicine* confirms the wisdom of Late Evan Bedford that this minor change in the mitral valve is very innocuous and is not the devil that it is made out to be by the echocardiographers and the many small and short term studies in the past. Barlow's original studies had thrown some light on this, but the present study is better conducted with better resources. Less than 2% of those with the so-called mitral valve prolapse syndrome get into any trouble. This is not higher than the ordinary population. This study clearly acquits MVP as the culprit. This should, at least, make our doomsday doctors wake up from their deep slumber! May the hapless victims of their attack breathe a sigh of relief. The study also points out to the significant overdiagnosis of the condition because of the faulty technique of echocardiography. Today cardiologists believe that echo is like a tomogram, and could be easily interpreted, howsoever done. Far from it, very far! The technique still is the key to correct diagnosis. In fact, I have described a new auscultatory method of diagnosing this condition even without the help of echocardiogram.

Many a person suffers because of bad technique. I have seen patients being angiogrammed with an echo diagnosis of thinning of the ventricular wall (due to silent infarcts etc.), while the fault was the original technique. Like the abdominal scans throwing up lots of young women with ovarian cysts of the diameter of a millimeter, creating the scare of cancer and then surgery, echocardiograms have made life miserable for quite a few in society. The above study in the NEJM could not have been timelier.

Even the king of sciences, physics, is not without such fallacies. Recently Richard Marsdon, Harvard astronomer, came up with his computer data that on the 26th October 2028, at 12.10 p.m. Central time in America there would circle the earth an asteroid of the size of a mile diameter, at a distance of 30,000 miles from earth. This has a fifty-fifty chance of hitting the earth. This prediction was very scary indeed! Similar asteroid, half its diameter, had hit the earth millions of years ago. The dust that it threw up closed off the sun from the earth for months that not a blade of grass grew here and the dinosaurs disappeared from the earth. People then got so scary that they started making all the arrangements, including insurance policies, to be on the safer side. Two days later another equally great astronomer, Donald Yeoman of NASA, could get similar data on his computer. The only difference was that the asteroid would be circling at 6,00,000 miles away from the earth and that there would not be a ghost of a chance that it would hit the earth. Insurances were then cancelled and people breathed a sigh of relief! This is not called mistake in science, the latter word is a taboo in science. It is called uncertainty! Similar is the story of mitral valve prolapse syndrome. The greatest discovery of the twenty-first century would be the discovery of man's ignorance!

Further Reading

- Hegde BM. Echocardiography-Its role in Clinical Medicine. *Karnataka Med J.* 1983; 50:49–54.
- Editorial. Do epidemiologists cause epidemics? *Lancet* 1993;341:993–994
- Freed LA, Levy D, Levine RA, et al. Prevalence and clinical outcome of mitral-valve prolapse. *N Engl J Med.* 1999; 341:1–7.
- Gilan D, Bounanno FS, Joffe MM, et al. Lack of evidence of an association between mitral-valve prolapse and stroke in young patients. *N Engl J Med* 1999; 341: 8–13.
- Nishimura RA and McGoon MD. Perspectives of mitral-valve prolapse. *N Engl J Med* 1999; 341:48–50.
- Hegde BM. Auscultation for MVP. *Lancet* 1994; 344: 1446–47.
- Hegde BM. Mitralklappen-Prolaps. *German Medical Tribune* 1995; 17: 36.

CHAPTER 35

Ne Plus Ultra

The medical fraternity, aided and abetted by the giant pharmaceutical industry believes and propagates the idea that mankind cannot remain healthy and win over illnesses without regularly getting medical help and consuming medicines. They, together, have come to the conclusion that there is nothing beyond medicine and doctors. I am reminded of Sir Francis Bacon's projected "*System of Philosophy*", The Great Instauration (*Novum Organum* – 1620 AD), which also believed in similar logic about this world.

Before Columbus set sail across the Atlantic, the coat of arms of the Royal Family of Spain had been an *impressa,* depicting the Pillars of Hercules (these pillars of Hercules were so huge that when compared to the world's tallest twin towers of Kuala Lumpur, they would make the latter look like small toilets!) and the Straits of Gibraltar, with the motto, **NE PLUS ULTRA**. There was **"No More Beyond"**. It was the pride and glory of Spain that their country was the outpost of the world. When Columbus made his discovery (of the New World), Spanish Royalty thriftily did the only thing necessary: erased the negative, leaving the giant Pillars of Hercules now bearing the motto, **PLUS ULTRA**. There was **More Beyond**.

Many of the *"new philosophers"*, now called *"scientists",* led by Sir Francis Bacon, regarded these inscriptions to be very prophetic and significant. The Pillars were supposed to signify the passage of knowledge just like the sailors, who pass to and fro between these Pillars. Medical scientists of today seem to believe in that motto. They seem to believe that there is *NO MORE BEYOND* modern medicine, to keep man alive on this planet. The enormous funds that flow from the powerful pharmaceutical industry helps to keep this myth alive, despite many evidences to the contrary. It also reminds me of the farming industry where the petrochemical giants perpetuate the myth that mankind could never be fed adequately unless the farming industry depended on chemical fertilizers.

Both these premises are flawed. Modern science of particle physics shows that the human being is only a tiny part of this macrocosm. It is our consciousness, which makes us tick in tune with the universal consciousness. Human body is a dynamic organism constantly run by food and oxygen but, totally dependent on the outside world, its environment. Human being is not a machine like a timepiece run by a spring. He/she does not work in bits and pieces, as was thought by Rene Descartes, and follow the conventional science of deterministic predictability of Newton and Albert Einstein. On the contrary, it works as a whole (holistic view) following the new science of particle physics of Max Planck, Max Bohm, Werner Heisenbeg and Erwin Schrodinger.

In their effort to combine the sciences of conventional physics and modern quantum mechanics, present day physicists are trying to get the two together in their "Unified Field" theory. Curiously, this is exactly what the Indian wisdom proclaimed to the world "time out of mind," in their own inimitable style thus: "**the whole universe is the container (space) and the content is universal consciousness**". If that were so, every human being becomes a tiny bit of that universe; totally interdependent and interconnected. Same is the story of agriculture. It is also dynamic and depends,to a large extent, on the soil and the multitude of organisms that go to make the soil fertile. Chemical fertilizers, in the end, would only promote the growth of weeds and sap the soil of its inherent fertility, acquired through the host of microorganisms that inhabit the soil.

There is an awareness of this even in the developed west where some farmers are following the natural organic farming methods. Chemical drugs from the pharmaceutical industry have been responsible for the mushrooming of the "super bugs," the multi-drug resistant microorganisms, in almost all hospitals, threatening patient safety. I only hope that we will not come one full circle to the time of "*hospitalism"* of the nineteenth century Britain, where seriously ill patients went to the hospital only to go to meet their maker sooner than later and never to return home.

In this scenario, human body would eventually suffer illnesses because of drugs and interventions, and agriculture would grow lots of weeds in place of useful food. Good wholesome food is a vital prerequisite for good health, anyway. The clear writing is already on the walls. Earlier mankind takes note of the warning, the better for the future generations. Many farming lobbies in the west and a few thinking farmers in India have taken note of this to reverse the trend. Still, the pressure of the multi-billion dollar giant of the petrochemical industry, helped by our Cartesian reductionist scientists and the all too obliging media, is trying to keep the dangerous myth alive that chemical fertilizers and genetically modified seeds are our saviours! Genetically modified seeds could be a more dangerous unforeseen threat to mankind.

The analogy fits the medical world very correctly. Doctors, from the day one at the medical school, are being brainwashed to believe that the bio-medical model of man as a machine, made up of independent parts, the organs, needs periodic servicing by doctors, even when the machine seems to be working well, lest it should break down without prior warning in the future. In addition, they are made to believe that drugs and interventions are the be-all and the end-all of disease management. Most of the reductionist scientists in this field help perpetuate this myth. This mechanistic paradigm of man as a bio-medical model has been the milch cow of the drug industry and the technology vendors. Interventions, more so, in apparently healthy population and their sheer numbers, has been financially very rewarding to the medical fraternity and the hospital giants. Medical education seems to be totally under the grip of these manipulators.

The reality, however, is different. The human body is built with enough safety measures to keep it going as long as possible with the help of its environment. The key player in this self preserving and self-sustaining game seems to be the human mind, while the external environment is an important ally. All functions of the human body follow three rhythms – the ultradian, the circadian and, the infradian. Of these, the last happens beyond the twenty-four hours' cycle, whereas the former two follow the day (24 hrs cycle). The infradian rhythm is the one that is controlled by the external forces, the environment, to a greater extent compared to the former two. In this context, I would like to mention the recent finding that the woman's menstrual cycle, a twenty eight days cycle, depends basically on the effect of the moons' gravitational force on the cortical cells of the brain to initiate and maintain the rhythm. This was proclaimed by Ayurveda thousands of years ago thus:

"*Kujendu hetu Prathimaasaarthavam*"
(Moon is the cause of monthly bleeding)

Ancient Indian science also proclaims that if one could keep one's mind (consciousness) tranquil, one could remain healthy until death. The modern science of particle physics agrees with this concept. The ground reality also supports this premise. Recent studies, many of them very large and prospective to have very high confidence levels, have shown that the human mind is one of the root causes of illnesses. Destructive hostility (hatred) has been shown to be the most important risk factor for heart attacks, while frustration and depression seem to be the real culprits in cancer and anger in haemorrhagic stroke. These cannot be the sole causes, but they are the prime-movers. Positive attitude has been shown to increase one's life span by five to seven years! In short, it is not what one eats that eventually kills one, but what eats one seems to be the main culprit.

One could also draw parallels from auditing many of our drug and technology interventions. When doctors went on strike in Israel recently and in Saskatchewan and Los Angels country in the past, mortality and morbidity fell down significantly. Routine screening and intervening in healthy men, in a milestone, long-term, prospective study, compared to non-intervention but with simple change of life style, did show significantly higher death and disability rates in the former. Interventions like coronary bypass surgery and angioplasty in symptomatic individuals, repeated breast scans using mammography, long-term hormone replacement therapy in postmenopausal women and, even routine long-term ingestion of vitamins and calcium supplements have only resulted in more morbidity and in some cases higher mortality. Even much hyped (and also lucrative) business of long-term blood pressure and sugar controlling drugs, as also the cholesterol lowering drugs, did not have the desired and predicted benefits!

"Time has come", the Walrus said, taking the oysters for a walk on the beach eventually to make a meal of them, to distract their attention "to talk of many things; cabbages and kings; of shoes and the polishing wax". Time has come for the medical fraternity to realize that, like the Walrus, the pharmaceutical and technology lobbies, assisted by the Cartesian reductionist scientists, might only be taking us for a walk up the garden path to make their tills moving. It is time doctors woke up before it is too late. Let us allow the new generation of medical students to think freely without the shackles of the wrong knowledge their textbooks contain. The existing knowledge would only make them status-quoists, following the footsteps of their forefathers. "Knowledge advances", said Karl Popper, "not by repeating known facts, but by refuting false dogmas." We have to refute the myth that the human body is a machine working in bits and pieces like a time clock. I was shocked recently to know that even medical textbooks, at least the majority of them, are written with the help of drug company finances. Less said about the research being financed by these companies the better. Even the best of journals had to retract papers. Drug lobby could easily doctor the research data to "see in research what they want to see".

In conclusion, let me remind the reader that there is a whole new world of medical science waiting to be rediscovered like the "gems of purest ray serene the dark unfathomed caves of ocean bear." Ayurveda, the mother of all medical wisdoms, has vital treasures, both for promoting health and correcting illness. Mind, shown earlier to be the kingpin in the game of human wellness or otherwise, occupies the pride of place in that holistic system. There are other medical care delivery systems as well. A judicious mix of the best in all these systems, along with the hi-tech modern technological medicine for emergency care, would not only benefit mankind, but also make medical facility available for the poorest of the poor. ***There is more beyond modern medicine – PLUS ULTRA.***

FURTHER READING

- Procedings of the WHOLE PERSON HEALING conference in Washington DC during the week 14th through 17th March 2005. rroy@psu.edu

CHAPTER 36

Woman, Moon and Menstruation

What a combination? We have studied in human physiology that a woman starts monthly bleeding from the time of menarche only to stop when she attains menopause. Where does the moon in the sky come into this picture? Naturally, by now you have concluded that I am about to write scientific fiction! Far from it; very, very far from it. You are in for a rude shock if you choose to read on. Most of us are like men inside a cave, enjoying the shadows inside and studying them, trying to give our own explanations and argue about it and be satisfied to agree to disagree. But, said Plato, in his celebrated book *The Republic,* classed among some of the best writings in the history of western literature, even though, in a manner of speaking, Plato was a European pagan, that there is another class of men. The latter he calls the philosophers:

> **And is not the love of learning,
> the love of wisdom, that is philosophy.**
>
> —Plato, *Republic Book I*

This book, *The Republic,* is now classed a shade higher than such great classics like Cicero's *De Republica,* St. Augustine's *City of God,* and Thomas More's *Utopia.* None of our intellectuals would then question the statements in that book. Plato says that progress comes from those daring people who go out of the cave to study things in the real sunlight. When they have done that study it is their duty to go back inside the cave to tell their peers about their experience.

One such great philosopher was Varahamihira, an Indian pagan, in the court of King Vikramaditya (lived around 100 BC). Varahamihira was considered to be one of the nine gems of Vikramaditya's court, the others included such great scholars like the peerless poet Kalidasa. Varahamihira was only Mihira when he joined the court. When the king had his first son, the court astrologers sat to decide on the future of the heir only to come up with the good omen that the child would live long to get name and fame for the kingdom. Mihira, who also was in the gathering, was perplexed, as his own calculations showed that the boy would die very young and would never become king at all. In addition, he also knew how the boy would die—to be killed by a wild boar! Mihira had the courage to oppose the great astrologers of the court in an open assembly. Everyone was shocked to hear this.

The King, visibly perturbed, gave Mihira one more chance to calculate. He came up with the same conclusions. King then ordered that if this does not come true Mihira's head should be cut off. He also made sure that all precautions were taken to protect the child. The inevitable happened and the child died as predicted soon afterwards despite human efforts by the great King. The King Vikramaditya decorated Mihira with many honours and then on he was called Varahmihira (Varaha-wild boar). The following stanza is from one of Varahamihira's great books on astrology.

Kujenduhetu pratimaasaarthavam

—*Varahamihira*

(Because of the Moon's control on the woman's body, she bleeds regularly once in twenty-eight days.)

I am sure, by now, you will have started to laugh within yourselves thinking that I am getting into the realm of superstition and mysticism. Be that as it may, let us look at the latest 2001 edition of the Cecil's *Textbook of Medicine*. In the present environment in our medical schools this American book would be valued more than The *Republic* (if ever the students have heard of Plato—they would have heard of Pluto, though) with the Damocles sword of examinations hanging precariously above their necks! As a student I had not read Plato myself. In fact, all that I learnt as a student helped me only to pass examinations, an important pre-requisite though. After passing I had to unlearn to relearn again the real life medicine. Cecil's book would also be admitted as evidence in an American court of law. Now read on the extract from that book (page 1202) on the physiology of menstruation:

"The pituitary has an intrinsic rhythm of small amplitude with a frequency of every two to ten minutes. Superimposed on this intrinsic rhythm is a rhythm caused by the pulsatile release of hypophysiotropic releasing factors, with or without the withdrawal of a corresponding inhibitory factor. Rhythms that are shorter than a day are referred to as ultradian rhythms. The next layer of rhythmicity is the circadian rhythm, i.e., rhythms with approximately 24-hour periodicity. These rhythms are usually synchronized with the 24-hour period by a periodic environmental cue such as dark-light cycle. The supra-chiasmatic nucleus functions as a circadian pace maker and receives light-induced electrical impulses from the retina via the retino-ophthalmic tract, finally transmitting those impulses to the pineal gland, where they are converted to hormonal signals. **Signals for a rhythm with a periodicity longer than 24 hours, i.e., an infradian rhythm, include the gravitational influence of the moon, which gives rise to the menstrual cycle.**"

There are a lot of things that we do not get to know when we rely only on our five senses only. To say that man's life on this planet is not at all influenced by celestial bodies is nothing short of arrogance of the first order that is unbecoming of a good scientist. One can say that astrology, as a science, is not accurate in predicting the future. No other science is accurate either. Do we not know the "butterfly effect" of Edward Lorenz? Science has been predicting the unpredictable all along. If one becomes humble, the sign of good education, one quickly realizes the importance of wisdom in contradistinction to knowledge. I am not an astrologer but I strongly feel that astrology plays a vital role in psychotherapy. There is a whole lot of literature on Ayurvedic Astrology that has been studied extensively even by westerners. Now that I have verbatim quoted the Cecil's textbook of Medicine above to give credibility to the ancient wisdom of India, I am sure even our hard-to-please scientists would agree that moon controls the menstrual cycle through its gravitational force.

There are many other actions inside the human body that the gravitational force of the moon could control. If billions of tons of water could shift from one part of the ocean to another due the gravitational pull of the moon in high and low tides, what about the human body, which is predominantly water? Many newer details about this are being unraveled everyday by scientific methods. I am grateful to my dear friend, Dr TI Radhakrishnan, FRCP(Edin.), a Queen's Square trained neurologist, that drew my attention to the latest edition of the Cecil's textbook. He has mounted a new study under his guidance to find out a scientific method to know the exact time of birth so that the astrological charts could be more accurate in future. I am awaiting the results with bated breath.

Our astrologers also should wake up from their slumber to admit that all that they have learnt so far need not be the whole truth and nothing but the truth. Science is change and we should strive to apply the latest scientific methods to verify our ancient claims and prove to the world their good qualities, if any. Let the scientific community rise to the occasion. Those of us who are in search of the truth could go on and try to unravel the mystery that is the human body and its marvels. Science is curiosity organized with a pinch of logical skepticism added. Results could be positive or negative. Ours shall only be the effort and the result is not in our hands. Long live true scientific temper for the good of humanity.

FURTHER READING

- *Cecil's Textbook of Medicine.* 2001 edition. Page 1202.
- Ali M. A Soulless Science. *J Integrative Medicine* 1997; 1: 1–6.

CHAPTER 37

Critical Care: More Things Not to Do

> **And is not the love of learning the love of wisdom, which is philosophy?**
>
> —Plato, *Republic, Book One*

More than ninety per cent of the American health care budget goes to keep patients alive in critical care units during the last ten days of their lives. This takes a heavy toll of the budget for health care elsewhere. To give a telling example, the money needed to keep a child alive in the terminal stage of leukaemia with bone marrow transplants would be equal to the amount needed to keep one thousand pregnant women healthy during their pregnancy as well as their infants' care for one year after delivery. This audit brought forth the Oregon Law that states that "no child would get a bone marrow transplant for leukaemia at the tax payer's cost." Although this started a lot of debate initially, right now seven other States in the US follow the same law.

Modern hi-tech medicine is a must for emergency care although its validity in chronic illnesses is seriously questioned. When a patient has trauma or any other acute catastrophic illness, we have to, per force, do our best even though the knowledge in that field is equivocal. That does not mean that any technology or drug should be used without proper audit even in the emergency situation. Many of the audits done so far have not yielded encouraging results. More alarming is the false propaganda of the sellers of drugs and technology in medicine. One European study reported in the *British Medical Journal* showed that only **6%** of the company literature is based on true scientific findings and the rest is only falsehood and mystery to sell their wares!

Let us take the Coronary Care Units as an example. First started in the Kansas City in 1962, they mushroomed all over the world and have even reached the far corners of the third world. The conventional coronary care units have been shown to have made no change in the mortality of acute myocardial infarction. The prevailing wisdom at that time was that the cause of death in acute MI is the arrhythmias. If one could monitor them for the first few days and treat quickly one could save countless lives. It looked so attractive that everyone got on to the bandwagon without critically evaluating them. Technology companies made enormous business in the bargain. In fact, one study, the Mather's study in Sheffield and Bristol, showed that marginally higher deaths occurred in those admitted to the CCUs while the Chief took rounds.

CCUs have now changed to ambulance coronary care units doling out thrombolytics at the onset of an acute MI claiming to save millions every year! Again it may be a statistical mirage! The first six hundred patients discharged from such emergency thromblysis did show marginally reduced in-hospital mortality only to be compensated more than adequately by post-discharge mortality in the next six months at home or work place, compared to those that did not get the benefit of the immediate thrombolysis. Then came the era of the TPA and the story is clear to all the readers by now.

Now if one talks to the divine interventionalists they would think that thrombolysis alone is no better than placebo unless it is combined with urgent post-infarction angioplasty and/or bypass surgery. Angioplasties have undergone remarkable changes. The old generation still believes in conventional angioplasty while the newer pundits think that simple plasty is useless unless one uses the drug eluting stents. Long term audits have not shown any one of these in good light. More dangerous and glaring is the recent audit on immediate post-infarction bypass surgery. The latter is shown to increase the fatal stroke rate to go up four fold in those that undergo immediate bypass. The study also showed that the greatest risk for fatal stroke now is **getting admitted, after a heart attack, to a coronary care unit with an attached bypass set up!**

Recent audits of the per capita mortality of those that were seriously injured in the Vietnam War vis-à-vis those of the Falklands war did show the large gap in our knowledge of managing acute trauma. Even fluid replacement is now in serious trouble with our limited understanding of the physiology of fluid loss. The "dry theorists" who lost out to the "wet theorists," that claimed supremacy of the drop per drop replacement of the lost fluid in the past, seem to have a valid point. This is discussed in greater detail elsewhere in the book.

The ill-understood physiology of DIC still makes us do things wrongly for those ill-fated DIC patients. The role of the gut wall in starvation in the immune system function of the victim needs further study before we embark on large scale parenteral feeding. The much touted Swan-Ganz catheter to measure the internal pressures has fallen by the way side having been shown to have sent millions to meet their maker prematurely in the last decade or two after its introduction. There are many, many more such uncritical critical care in use these days that cry for serious audit in the best interests of our gullible patients. To do or not to do is the biggest dilemma facing doctors today.

Drugs are no different. While there are six guidelines for hypertension management, all of them put together, include only 39% of hypertensives in their inclusion criteria. The remaining majority of 61% do not have any guidelines except intelligent guessing by the wise doctors! Where then is our evidence based medicine? Many more such things are discussed in this book in other chapters, anyway. "One of the essential qualities of the clinician is interest in humanity, for the secret of patient care is caring for the patient," wrote Francis Weld Peabody (1882–1927). How very true, indeed! Let us care for our patients even when they are in the critical care area.

Men are "vain authorities who can resolve nothing."

—Michel de Montaigne, *The Essays, (II-13)*

Further Reading

- Hegde BM. To do or not to do. *Kuwait Medical Journal 2002*
- Roach GW, Kanchuger M, Mangano CM, et al. Adverse cerebral outcomes after coronary bypass surgery. *N Engl J Med* 1996;335:1857–63.
- Tuffs HA. Only 6% of drug advertising material is supported by evidence. *BMJ* 2004; 328: 485.
- Spodick DH. Swan-Ganz catheter. *Chest* 1999; 115: 857–858.
- Selenes OA, McKhann GM. Coronary artery bypass and the brain. *N Engl J Med* 2001; 334: 451–452.
- Hegde BM. *Heart Manual* 2003. UBSPD, New Delhi-5. India.

CHAPTER 38

Antibiotic Crisis – A Time Bomb?

Nearly seventy years ago, when Alexander Fleming and Prof Florey discovered a moldy growth on their culture plates to be a powerful antibiotic, penicillin, a new era began in medicine. The predictions then were, as usual, that the end of man's fight against germs on this planet is drawing closer. Like all other predictions in linear science this one has also been belied. Doctors have been predicting the unpredictable all these years. That in itself is not bad! But we are now facing a new and formidable threat in that many of the germs that were initially sensitive to antibiotics have now become resistant and threaten to annihilate man from this planet. One example would suffice. One common germ, the streptococcus, was the most sensitive germ to be killed by penicillin. While 95% of these germs could be easily killed by penicillin to begin with, today 95% of the same are resistant to penicillin.

The history of this universe is very closely connected to human births and deaths, but illnesses do change history much more dramatically compared to the former two. The black death due to plague in Europe in the sixteenth century, the white death—so called because it killed most people with extreme anemia and mostly young adolescents in particular—of tuberculosis, have been the greatest tragedies of mankind. Tuberculosis still eludes a cure despite our euphoria after the advent of antibiotics against the germ *Mycobacterium tuberculosis*. In fact, it has become much more rampant and dangerous now that AIDS abets and assists the former to ravage human life.

Tuberculosis has assumed a different form these days because of the changing circumstances. Historical milestones of tuberculosis include the hunchbacks of Egyptian mummies, the phthisis (wasting) of the Greeks, and the English consumption of the lay public. Most diseases respected wealth and status to a certain extent, but plague and TB did play truant even with the rich and the famous from time to time.

The gravity of the situation is such that the Royal College of Physicians of London organized a meet to discuss the *Clinical Implications of Anti-microbial Resistance* on the 28th February 2001. It has been estimated that around 15,000 people die in that small country every year from infections against which no antibiotic is effective. Such of those germs that are resistant to most antibiotics are called the *super bugs* and, as of now, we have no defense against them. One of the biggest hospitals in that country, Portsmouth Hospitals NHS Trust, has been forced to shut down most of its operating theatres last summer because of *super bugs* there. At the Queen Alexandra Hospital, the orthopedic surgeons could not perform any operation around that time. Another leading authority in the field, Professor Hugh Pennington of Aberdeen University, feels that the next big problem would be that of drug resistant tuberculosis. They had an outbreak of TB in Scotland recently, traced to a traveling family. He also feels that the Russian prisons have many inmates who have drug resistant TB without proper treatment. Since TB does not respect geographic borders this time bomb might explode anytime anywhere!

The usual thinking in the West was that this kind of uncontrolled infectious disease scenario could exist only in the poor countries like India and sub-Saharan Africa. They are now in for a great shock. In a well researched book, *Betrayal of Trust: The Collapse of Global Public Health,* Laurie Garrett, from the USA, shows how the threat is not confined to the poor countries but, is greater in the West, basically because doctors there overprescribe antibiotics so that bacterial infections are becoming increasingly resistant to the most widely used antibiotics. She writes that "doctors who overprescribe antibiotics undermine the health care system by encouraging germs to become resistant." She is dead right there.

FURTHER READING

- Firth WJ. Chaos-Predicting the unpredictable. *BMJ* 1991;303:1565–68.
- Breathnach AS, de Ruiter A, Holdsworth GM, et. al. An outbreak of multi-drug resistant TB in a London teaching hospital. *J Hosp Infect.* 1998; 39: 111–117.
- Garrett L. *Betrayal of Trust-The collapse of the global public health.* 2000. New York, Herpion.

- Culpepper L, Froom J. Routine anti-microbial treatment for otitis media-is it necessary? *JAMA* 1997; 278: 1643–1645.
- Doolittle WF. You are what you eat: a gene transfer rachet could account for bacterial genes in eucaryocytic nuclear genomes. *Trends Genet.* 1998; 14: 307–311.
- Davies J. Inactivation of antibiotics and dissemination of resistance genes. *Nature* 1997; 389: 924.
- Handworth B. Maggots treat as they eat. *National Geographic Newsletter.* 2003, October 24th.
- Dormondy T. *The White Death.* 1999, Hambledon Press, London.
- Starfield B. Is US health care the best in the world? *JAMA* 2000; 284: 483–485.

CHAPTER 39

Needless Interventions in Medicine

"All that glitters is not gold" is an old, but true adage. Cardiac interventions, heading the list of many such interventions in modern medicine, have been hogging the limelight for the last three decades or so. Whereas they have a very definite role to play in palliating intractable pain and/or refractory left heart failure following a heart attack or crescendo angina, **they certainly do not have a role in patients who are asymptomatic, but have blocks in their coronary vessels with good left ventricular function.** I have been one of those hapless victims of a vilification campaign for having been saying this in last two decades.

More studies, on a larger number of patients, in contrast to the small studies done with funding from the instrument manufacturers, have demonstrated the real picture. These studies do not get read so widely by the people that matter the most—our practicing physicians—as many of the latter do not have the time and inclination to get deep into this dense forest of medical literature, where more than 35,000 new articles appear, in the innumerable bio-medical journals every month! It is, additionally, very difficult for the novice to get into this jungle of medical literature and actually distinguish the rose wood from firewood. That is the sole purpose of reiterating what I have been saying for years, with more evidence from newer studies, in this chapter.

Many other interventions have had similar stories. A glaring example would be that of the Swan-Ganz catheter that was being used literally in every patient in the intensive therapy unit and the Coronary Care Units. A recent study of some American hospitals revealed that the catheter itself could have caused nearly 100,000 deaths in four years! This has created a general awareness in the medical circles, and many have asked for a moratorium on the Swan-Ganz catheter.

There are many other interventions that have not been audited before being used on the gullible public, unlike the newer drugs that, per force, have to go through randomized controlled human trials, before being used in patients. There have been fatal errors in this procedure even in cases of drugs, the glaring example being milrinone in heart failure treatment.

There was a time when the inventors of a newer device insisted that they test it on themselves before using it on the hapless patients. A good example is that of Late Dr Lewis Dexter. In the year 1944, Lewis Dexter was studying renin in hypertensive patients. With his catheter in the inferior vena cava to get into the renal vein he wandered a bit further up above the diaphragm. To his dismay he found that his catheter had slipped into the lung of the patient. Dexter was sure that he had perforated the heart. He then did not know what to do! He put on the lights and asked the patient "Mr S..., How are you?" The patient said: "I look a hell of lot better than you look." Shocked that he must have punctured the heart, Dexter wrote the following paragraph in the case sheet that day, the 7th December 1944: "Then I was pretty sure that, having perforated the heart, it just sort of sealed itself off and [I] wondered what would happen when I pulled it out. So I closed my eyes and then pulled it out-nothing happened. And then...it was all over and I put a little Band-Aid on his entry wound and went and looked up the anatomy of the chest and figured I had gone into the pulmonary artery."

Dexter then discussed his adventure with Dr C Sydney Burwell, the dean of the Harvard Medical School at that time. The latter suggested that if Dexter could get to the pulmonary artery that easily, he could study congenital heart diseases in greater detail!

But Dexter wanted to put the catheter first into his own pulmonary artery to show to others that it was safe. He also wanted to do some exercise when he had the catheter inside him to verify that no harm could come to any patient from pulmonary artery catheterization. No one had done that before him. **He did not believe that he should subject anybody for a procedure that he himself would not be willing to undergo.** He asked one of his Fellows to place the catheter in his heart and pushed it to the pulmonary artery himself. He then gently sat up. Everyone was holding his or her breath and thought Dexter would have a cardiac arrest anytime! It was a time before defibrillators! Then he stood up. Nothing happened to him. He then skipped a bit and then proceeded to do vigorous exercise, recording all the changes in the heart during exercise. That is what we need in people wanting to sell technology without controlled studies. I hope people get the message.

A large study of 18,151 patients who underwent bypass surgery immediately after a heart attack or following an attack of crescendo angina (unstable angina) showed that they were nearly **four times more likely to have a subsequent stroke than those who did not have bypass surgery.** Death in these stroke patients following bypass surgery was much higher! **This study showed, in addition, that bypass surgery was the most important predictor of stroke** followed by past history of stroke, diabetes, and older age group. The most glaring finding of this study, about which I have written many times in the past, is that **the existence of an onsite catheterization laboratory facility was also a risk factor for subsequent stroke in those hapless patients with a heart attack admitted to such hospitals.**

This study did not show a statistically increased occurrence of stroke following angioplasty. Those wanting to sell angioplasty could use this as their marketing strategy. They cannot, however, escape the findings of another study that showed that "**angioplasty may lead to greater reduction in anginal pain compared to medical treatment but at a cost of more coronary artery bypass grafting...although all the randomized controlled trials done all over the world and published between 1979 and 1998 do not give enough data about death and subsequent revascularization, the trends so far DO NOT FAVOUR ANGIOPLASTY."**

Curiously, another study has shown that "initial angioplasty may complicate the bypass operation and may increase postoperative mortality and morbidity." An audit on an earlier study of bypass surgeries did show that in those without symptoms a **large majority of 84% recipients of bypass surgery did not get any survival benefits from their interventions.** Only 16% did get some small benefit. This study had audited a large number of such procedures, running to nearly 60,000.

Other studies in the past have also thrown light on the side effects of bypass surgery on the brain. These studies showed the incidence of stroke following bypass surgery to be anywhere between 1.5 to 5.2%, postoperative delirium to be 10–30%, and cognitive decline to range from 53% on discharge to 42% on a long-term basis.

One could go on and on, but that would take away the punch of this message which centers around coronary bypass surgery, the one intervention that is the till-mover of many fee-for-service hospitals, bringing glory and limelight for the star-performers.

As a rare exception, this particular procedure is a pain in the neck for only the rich, and does not, at the moment, bother the poor. In most cases, the latter are at the receiving end of every single illness, while the former are generally unaffected. Their body's repair wisdom and faith in their doctor's capacity to heal—the placebo effect—usually look after the poor, when they get coronary artery disease. They are the lucky ones, for a change. The scenario is not very different for many of the drugs used in chronic "doctor-thinks-you-have-a disease" syndromes like hyperlipidaemias, mild-moderate hypertension, and asymptomatic hyperglycaemia.

I better conclude this narration by quoting CD Naylor in his article in the *Archives of Internal Medicine* thus: "While journal editors have the responsibility to ensure that physicians have ready access to adequate summaries of clinical trials of preventive interventions, ensuring that patients have a similarly objective view of the results before embarking on therapy becomes the responsibility of the physician. Of note, in a hypothetical treatment decision, **79% of the patients stated that they would decline a lipid-lowering drug suggested by their physician after seeing the benefit expressed in an unflattering numeric format.**"

Time has come for openness. We cannot blame those who keep performing interventions left, right, and centre, as they know not that linear relations do not work in a dynamic system like the human body. Whereas coronary blocks start very early in life, the symptoms of ischaemic heart disease start at a much later date, after the body's compensatory mechanisms weaken with the burden of the ageing process. The four epicardial vessels pictured in the angiogram play a minor role, while the real culprits are the four million small perforating muscle arteries, which normally have an enormous capacity to dilate to accommodate extra blood on demand, called the coronary reserve. Unlike what the interventionalists think, the coronary block is not akin to a block in a rigid water pipe. The body's wisdom tries its best to compensate for arterial blocks by remodeling. It is also true that when the vessels are bad in one part of the body, the vessels elsewhere are equally bad. **The connection between heart attacks and brain attacks, seen above, is not surprising at all. In fact, it should have been expected in advance!**

There are many things in interventional medicine that we should not be doing, unless our backs are pressed to the wall. It is our moral obligation to bring this to the notice of our patients and let them take the final decision in any intervention, guided by us as partners in disease management. The time has come for partnership in patient care in place of paternalism.

FURTHER READING

- Hegde BM. Coronary revascularisation-time for reappraisal. *Proc Roy Coll Physi Edin* 1995; 26: 421–424
- Hegde BM. Need for change in medical paradigm. *Proc Roy Coll Physi Edin*. 1993; 23: 9–12
- Spodick DH. The Swan-Ganz catheter. *Chest* 1999; 115: 857–858
- Stein PD. Lewis Dexter, MD-The end of an era. *Circulation* 1996; 94: 229–230
- Mukyopadhyaya M. A biographical Sketch of Lewis Dexter. *Tex Heart Inst J* 2001; 28: 133–138
- Joesefson D. Early bypass surgery increases the risk of stroke. *BMJ* 2001; 323: 185
- Bucher HC, Hengstler P, Schindler C, and Guyatt GH. PTCA versus Medical treatment for non-acute coronary heart disease. *BMJ* 2000; 321: 73–77
- Kalaycioglu S, Sinci V, and Oktar L. CABG after successful PTCA. Is PTCA a risk for CABG? *Int Surg* 1998; 83: 190–193
- Yusuf S, Zucker D, Peduzzi P et al. Effect of CABG on survival. *Lancet* 1994; 344: 565–568
- Hornick P, Smith PL, Taylor KM. Cerebral complication following coronary bypass grafting. *Curr Opin Cardiol* 1994; 9: 670–679
- Selens OA and McKhann GM. Coronary Artery Bypass and the Brain. *N Engl J Med* 2001; 344: 451–453
- McCormack J and Greenhalgh T. Seeing what you want to see in research. *BMJ* 2000; 320: 1720–1723
- Anderson OK, Almgren T, Persson B, et al. Survival in treated hypertension. *BMJ* 1998; 317: 167–171
- Hux JE and Naylor CD. In the eye of the beholder. *Arch Intern Med* 1995; 155: 2277–2280
- Hegde BM. Chaos- a new concept in science. *J Assoc Physi India* 1996; 44: 167–168.

CHAPTER 40

Mothers, Babies, and Killer Diseases

> A mother is a mother still,
> The holiest thing alive...
>
> —*Coleridge*

A dedicated community nurse midwife in Hertfordshire County in England, Ethel Margaret Burnside, tried her best to reduce infant mortality in the early part of the last century, before the First World War, despite all drawbacks. She was known as the bicycle nurse as she did not have a car to go about. The meticulous records of every birth there, recorded in indelible ink in her best handwriting, gave new insight into the possible triggering factors of major killers like heart attacks, vessel blocks, high blood pressure, diabetes, etc. Of course, you would wonder as to the connection between the births and all these illnesses! Another equally tenacious researcher, Professor David Barker of the Southampton University, who was born in that County, chanced upon those records when he went in search of his sister's birth details. The records are the property of the archives now. They are not to be disclosed for another fifty years. Because of his sister's birth, David could access the records.

He tried to get all the medical records of those babies, now in their 80s and 90s, if alive, and also the death details of those who had already gone to meet their maker. Luckily, all this was possible in that country. Having obtained the details, David went on comparing their medical details with their birth details not knowing that he would stumble upon a serendipitous rare discovery. **Those babies that were born underweight were the ones that had premature heart attacks, diabetes, and vascular diseases, as well as other medical problems in later life.**

David went into greater details of these smaller than normal babies only to discover that they were born with very large placentae. He was able to fish out the details of the mothers' pregnancy of these babies as well, thanks to the efforts of Ethel mentioned earlier. Almost all the mothers of the babies that were born small with very large placentae came from either a very poor background where they did not have proper nutrition during the first trimester of pregnancy (when all the foetal organs get formed inside the womb) or had a rare disease called hyperemesis gravidarum—pregnancy vomiting—resulting in the mothers not taking in sufficient nutritious food. Maybe Nature, in its wisdom, tried to keep these babies alive inside the womb of a poorly fed mother by increasing the size of the placenta two to three fold to see that the baby gets adequate blood to somehow keep it going.

David Barker put the pieces of the jigsaw puzzle together and came up with his hypothesis that **underweight babies whose mothers were undernourished during pregnancy, especially the first trimester, do not have properly built organs like the heart, blood vessels, and the pancreas, which in later life, especially if the hapless off-springs put themselves in a food-plenty environment, could result in premature vascular damage, heart diseases, and diabetes.** Further studies by other researchers have now revealed that the iron pigment in mother's diet has a great bearing on the child's hippocampus major growth. Iron deficiency in pregnancy could bring forth children with less than adequate memory power.

Although the hypothesis was attractive, vested interests would not accept it without proof. David was lucky twice. He found out that a veterinary researcher in New Zealand was studying the same problem in ewes prospectively, and had come up with the data that if the mother is deliberately kept undernourished during the time of the formation of foetal organs, the foetus would either die in utero or the surviving foetus is kept alive by nature with the extra supply of blood to the growing foetus through a larger than normal placenta. This was the much needed support that David obtained for his serendipitous discovery using the Hertfordshire county retrospective data. David has helped similar studies in India at the Holdsworth Memorial Hospital, Mysore, where similar records are available. This hospital was founded in the name of a Hertfordshire county nurse whose husband kept the memory of his late wife alive in a city where his wife worked as a missionary nurse.

This is a great lesson for developing countries where the majority of women, especially from the socially deprived classes, have poor nutrition during pregnancy. Rich ones also might not eat well due to pregnancy vomiting or due to the new fad of thin figure as a beauty symbol. This could be one of the important contributing factors for premature diabetes, heart attacks, and high blood pressure in young people these days. The truth is more obvious in those individuals who migrate to western countries or to the Gulf to earn their bread, from the third world. They inadvertently put themselves into a food-plenty atmosphere there. This kind of **food-gene mismatch** results in their becoming diabetics early in life. Deformed small blood vessels also lead to premature clogging and raise blood pressure early on in life. The additional stress of present day living adds to the burden and results in premature death and disability due to heart attacks. The conventional, much-touted risk factors have very little to do with this newer disease profile as is very clearly shown by many studies of Asian immigrants in the West.

The moral of the story is that pregnant mothers need very good nutritious food all through pregnancy, but more so in the first three months of pregnancy. Our knowledge of pregnancy and child birth has advanced so much more to the point that we now know that prenatal consciousness is influenced by the environment in which the pregnant woman lives. A tranquil home, good relations, and good work environment could bring forth a bright child. The child starts to learn right from day one inside the mother's womb. Suffice it to say that our lives depend very much on our prenatal life in our mother's womb. Future mothers must have this knowledge *lest they take their pregnancy nutrition very lightly*. We could look forward to a world of good humans if our pregnant mothers are well cared for.

> **One of the essential qualities of the clinician is interest in humanity, for the secret of the care of the patient is in caring for the patient.**
>
> —*Francis Weld Peabody, 1881–1927*

Further Reading

- David Barker. *Mothers, Babies and killer Diseases.* BMA publications 1997.

CHAPTER 41

Science and the Tower of Babel

> Knowledge is the process of piling up facts; wisdom lies in their simplification.
>
> —*Martin H Fisher*

There is now a new controversy around a much-hyped pain killer, the COX 2 inhibitor, sold at a phenomenal price all over the world. While a reputed National Institute of Cancer study in the US revealed that this pain killer was responsible for a large number of heart attacks and strokes in those that take it on a long term basis to suppress pain, the manufacturer refuses to believe that report and is not recalling the drug from the market. The remedy suggested is that the authorities in the US send emails to all doctors to refrain from prescribing the drug.

The media, on the contrary, is going to town painting this drug as the best pain killer. I feel the media should do a bit of soul searching before publishing articles on health and drugs: some of them are even dangerous to read. I believe magazines will not sell in the market if they write the truth that "science works slowly and many a time gets things wrong, before it gets it right, if ever it gets them right!" So, what we see is a new drug to cure cancer, a cure-all for sex problems, a quick fix for obesity, etcetera. With all the fanfare, cancer is yet to be cured, sex is still an enigma, and obesity is threatening to be an epidemic. The war on any one of them is anything but won!

The problem with science is the language barrier between various subspecialists. They never can understand one another and will not even sit together to talk. This reminds me of the story in Genesis, where the people of Babel wanted to build a tower to reach heaven. God, in His wisdom, stopped this project by giving people different languages. Since they could not communicate, the tower could not be built! In science this is the reason why they are not able to get things right. Specialization and reductionism has killed any real progress. David Ewing Duncan of the San Francisco Chronicle calls this the bio-Babel. The First Law of Thermodynamics says that "anything that divides eventually disappears." Today science has divided so much that in medical science we have right ear specialists and left ear ones that do not seem to see eye to eye on any ear!

My writings in the last forty odd years have not been welcome in the lay media, although many have been published reluctantly. When I am invited to speak in scientific meetings some in the audience give me an impression that I am "Genghis Khan come to represent the tyrants view to the world peace summit" or I am like "Gavin Newsom trying to defend gay marriages at the John Birch Society." Drug companies have become a Frankenstein, which is difficult to put back in the bottle: some of their annual profits could buy up the US government. Having tasted blood they are not going to keep quiet and listen to sermons from anyone. When some of the "thought leaders" in our profession deliver their talks in "scientific" meetings with beautiful company-made slides to illustrate their points of view, they again talk a different language like the people of Babel. They mean goodbye when they say hello.

Writing in her excellent book *The Truth about Drug Companies: How they Deceive Us and What we Could Do about It,* the author, Marcia Angell, who teaches at Harvard, gives a graphic description of drug company deception. In another book, *Overdo$ed America,* a family physician in the US, John Abramson, cites instances of how the medical world is taken to the market place to the detriment of the hapless suffering humanity. Eric Schlosser, writing about the second book, has this to say and it says it all: "Some of the nation's worst drug dealers aren't peddling on street corners, they are occupying corporate suites. Overdo$ed America reveals the greed and corruption that drive the health care costs skyward and threaten the public health. Before you $ee a doctor, you should read this book."

What is the remedy? Scientists should try to be humble and try to understand one another. Reductionism does not work in dynamic systems of this universe and never works in the dynamic human body. There is always the danger of the "butterfly effect" in most of the interventions we doctors attempt. If we understand one another there is a good hope that we will be able to "cure rarely, comfort mostly, but console always." This has been the motto of medicine in the past. Those days should come back and most of the divine interventions to palliate symptoms should give way to more mundane things like life-style changes of the population that save more lives than all the hi-tech stuff that we talk about put together. The media goes to town with technology to spread the false message far and wide.

An audit recently showed that life-style changes, education, better sanitary conditions, and affluence reduce the burden of most diseases and, in fact, doctors and hospitals have only added to the burden. The reduced mortality in Israel when doctors went on strike, the Institute of Medicine report in the US, which showed that doctors and hospitals are the third most important cause of death and disability, and adverse drug reactions, should awaken scientists of all hues from their deep slumber.

The bio-technologists should realize that what happens between molecules, atoms and cells need not replicate in organs and definitely not in organisms. The debate about ultimate medical care should be holistic and should never be Balkanized among the different castes of scientists. The "star performers" in the field of medicine and surgery should be humble enough to audit their results on a long-term basis. Whereas Philadelphia did nearly eight times more bypass surgeries compared to Ontario, cities with identical populations, in the immediate post heart attack scenario, at the end of a year and five years there were equal number of people alive in both places in this group. This should make anyone sit up and take notice. The time has come to forget our differences and sit together using the same language to talk of the future of science and technology. Mere economic growth is not true progress. True progress depends on progressive thinking in a healthy way in society with all people speaking the same language.

> **There are few men who dare to publish to the world the prayers they make to Almighty God.**
>
> —Michel de Montaigne

Further Reading

- Editorial. Drug Company influence on medical education in USA. *Lancet* 2000; 356: 781–83.
- John Abramson. *Overdo$ed America,* 2004. Harper Collins, New York.
- Marcia Angell. *The Truth About Drug Companies.* 2004, Random House, New York.555555555555

CHAPTER 42

Scientific Superstitions

> *I don't give them hell. I just tell the truth and they think it is hell.*
>
> —*Harry S Truman*

The word *superstition* is used here to mean reverence for, or belief in, principles which are not worthy of worship. Scientific temper is to have curiosity about anything and everything and must not accept anything without getting into the core of the matter, using accepted methods of scrutiny. One must have this scientific temper in any field of human endeavour lest humankind should fall back into the valley of 'illogicalism'. However, in science today, there are many areas where blind faith in certain principles has led us astray and landed science in a mess. I shall confine this chapter to medical science in particular but it could be extended to other areas as well. Why is science in this mess today?

I am reminded of the story of the Tower of Babel referred to in an earlier chapter. In the Book of Genesis this story stands out for its moral value. When the people of Babel wanted to erect a tower to reach heaven, God, in His wisdom, must have been concerned. He decides to give the people of Babel different languages so that they could not understand each other and consequently, the Tower was never built. This is where science is today. We have divided scientific activity into narrower and narrower specialties that today a physicist does not understand a chemist, and abiologist does not understand either of them.

Medical science is in a total mess since it began riding piggyback on the natural sciences in the 12th Century AD. It is still deep into the conventional laws of deterministic predictability, even though it deals with a dynamic human system that does not follow those rules even for a second. We have been, therefore, predicting the unpredictable future of hapless patients and making life miserable for them. Anything that divides eventually disappears, avers one of the Laws of Thermodynamics. Unless specialists come together to understand each other, science has no future so long as we have different languages for different people like the people of the city of Babel.

This above statement has been more than ratified by recent studies in the west. The IOM report in the US has shown that doctors and hospitals are the third most important cause of death and that Adverse Drug Reactions (ADR) are the fourth! Another European study of five countries showed that where there are more doctors there is less health and vice versa. A recent doctors' strike in Israel brought the death and disability rates remarkably down during the strike period only to return to their original levels after doctors went back to work. Interventions in *healthy* people to avoid later catastrophes have been disastrous in the long run.

Risk Factor Hypothesis

This has been the biggest myth in medicine. Consider the sites designated to clean up hazardous waste. The calculated risk of someone getting cancer from those sites is 1 in 10,000 or more. The risk is so small that it would take a study of at least 500 million people (twice the US population) to prove such a small risk. One can never be proved right or wrong in such a situation. Some of the more famous unproven risks are the ones that are flaunted on the public day in and day out! We are only assessing relative risks and not *absolute risk!* In this scenario anything could be a risk factor. Wearing a brassiere all day long could be a great risk for breast cancer! Biological plausibility is the only certainty in this area. However, one of the greatest worries for the lay people (who can read these health magazines) is this silly risk factor hypothesis—a superstition indeed.

Statistical Significance

The *p-value* indicates the probability that a statistical association is a fluke. The smaller the p-value the better. If it is below 0.05 there is a less than 5% chance of your association being a fluke and a 95% chance that it is true; a 95% confidence interval. However, the p-value is immutable.

If it is above 0.05, one could manage to fix it to show better results. There are methods to do that, but we will not go into that here. Medical science, therefore, is only a statistical science and not a true science to be totally relied upon.

Randomised Controlled Studies

Claimed to be the last best thing to have happened to medical research, randomized controlled studies have been the biggest superstition of all times. We compare two cohorts of humans matched by body mass index and a few known phenotypic characteristics. The cohorts are, therefore, supposed to be identical. But a human being is more than just a phenotype. A "Whole" human is genotype, phenotype, and consciousness. Unless one gets the total picture, time evolution can never be predicted. Time evolution does not depend on partial knowledge of the initial state of an organism, but on the *whole* knowledge. Under the circumstances, controlled studies have no meaning at all. To cap it, time evolution might not keep pace with minor changes in the initial state of an organism over time. This is the main reason why most, if not all drugs, in the long run have done more damage than good to patients, emerging as the fourth important cause of death in the US.

Blind Extrapolation

Extrapolating controlled study data to patients is another superstition. There are no controlled studies of many drugs used in combination, while in reality patients often take many tablets simultaneously. Controlled studies have been done for short periods of time, rarely up to five years, but patients take drugs for decades. Worse still is extrapolating animal studies to humans. Even though this practice has burnt our fingers many a time in the past, the superstition continues unabated. One of the provocations to write this chapter is a patient that I saw recently. She was a middle aged physician's wife who was on 28 tablets and daily insulin injections at the same time! I do not think that there has been a controlled study of this kind of combination anywhere in the world to date. God only knows what these drugs do in tandem and to one another within the human body.

Faith in Drug Company Sponsored Research

Two recent books by eminent authors in the US reiterated what I had been writing for decades. Marcia Angell, the former editor in chief of the *New England Journal of Medicine,* in her celebrated book *The Truth About Drug Companies* published by Random House, and John Abramson in his classic *Overdo$ed America* published by Harper Collins, exposed the dangerous scenario of the drug company fraud. Still better is the book *Health Myths Exposed* by Shane Ellison. Despite the many glaring instances of fraud, drugs are still being marketed by companies under various garbs. Doctors are being bought over by these companies and the so-called "thought leaders" on the company payroll are the real culprits in making the gullible public and the medical profession believe in their wisdom to pontificate.

Research Fraud

Disease clusters and Texas sharpshooters, data dredging, the mix-master technique—otherwise called meta-analysis—baked biological plausibility, picking the right animal species to show positive results, maximizing dosage, and the final doctoring and sexing up of data are all regular practices in medical research. Peer review is another one of those untested methods to authenticate one's research data. I have not been able to understand how peer reviewing could be fool proof! Many of the reputed journals also have editorial policies that might assist in these processes. To cite one example, many a time any *original* study is accompanied by an editorial by a guest editor. Most, if not all, of these breed of wise people are on the payroll of the drug company that funded the research in the first place! The new *avatar* of drug trials in developing countries is another great fraud on the gullible public. These CROs (Clinical Research Organisation) are only brokers who get drugs studied in developing countries to make huge profits for themselves. They entice doctors in those countries with relatively comfortable perks compared to their otherwise limited earning capacity. One could only imagine the results in this setting. Of course, the trial results are the property of the sponsoring company and are published by them.

With this background in mind, medical research becomes highly suspect. The most important facts have yet to be discovered. With nearly forty thousand bio-medical journals in the field and new information coming out at a phenomenal pace of 7% per month, there have been very few, if any, refutative research data, which could take knowledge forward in any area. Most of the data have been repetitive. I have not touched upon the remedy for this serious illness, which requires thinking people to come together to stop this menace. There are moves afot in this direction led by Prof Rustom Roy, the father of nanotechnology at the Penn State University in the US, who has now started a group called the *whole person healing group*.

> **If data have been cooked and the results plausible, there is no way peer review can catch the fraud.**
>
> —*Arnold S Relman*
> Then editor-in-chief of New England Journal of Medicine in the Washington Post, May 16th, 1989.

FURTHER READING

- Firth WJ. Chaos-predicting the unpredictable. *BMJ* 1991; 303: 1565–1568.
- Starfield B. Is the US medicine best in the world? *JAMA* 2000; 284: 483–485.
- Smith R. Doctors going on strike could be good for society. *EMJ* 2003; 326: 456.
- Milloy S. *Science without Sense.* 1993. CATO Institute, Washington DC.
- Hegde BM. To do or not to do. *J Indian Academy of Clin Med* 2002; 3(3): 236–239.
- Packer M, Carver JR, Rodeheffer RJ, et al. Effect of oral milrinone on mortality in severe chronic heart failure. The PROMISE research group. *N Engl J Med.* 1991; 325: 1468–1475.
- Eaton L. Editor claims drug companies have a parasitic relationship with journals. *BMJ* 2005; 330: 9–10.
- Altman K. The scandal of poor medical research. *BMJ* 1994; 308: 283–284.
- Campbell EG, Louis KS, Blumenthal S. Looking the gift horse in the mouth. *JAMA* 1998; 279: 995–999.

CHAPTER 43

Uncertainty is the only Certainty

Richard Smith, the then editor of the *British Medical Journal,* was lamenting, in one of his recent editorials, about the poor communication skills of doctors in general and their incapacity to deal with uncertainties in medicine. Doctors have been predicting the unpredictable outcomes of their interventions to patients all along. Time evolution does not depend on patchy knowledge of the initial state of a patient. This myth of future predictions is at the root of patients losing confidence in their doctors. If one is well and healthy at any given time, it is because of *chance:* if, on the contrary, one is unwell it is still because of *chance.* In fact, the word *chance* simply signifies God without His signature being affixed.

The answer to this dilemma is to teach medical students in training that doctors, like everyone else, are fallible and could make mistakes, and should try to learn from these mistakes to avoid repetition. Being honest about the mishap, and sharing one's joys and sorrows with the patient could ease the situation and enhance communication. The crux of the healing process is the coming together of two human beings—the one who thinks she/he is ill or imagines that she/he is ill and the other in whom the former has confidence. This coming together of two human beings with mutual trust is the summit of medicine from where all other aspects like diagnosis, therapy, future management, etcetera flow. It is here that the patient gains confidence in his/her doctor.

Sincerity, honesty, and being open about the hollowness of the myth that the medical profession could bring back people from the jaws of death would create a better rapport between the doctor and the patient. Technology, in the last half century, has deified the medical profession sending wrong signals to patients to expect the impossible from their doctors—one of the reasons for the burgeoning consumer suits in the west against the medical profession. This has transformed the holy doctor-patient relationship into that of a seller and a buyer, resulting in the market forces uprooting medical ethics. "Cure rarely, comfort mostly, but console always" was good Hippocratic advice. It is not what the doctor tells the patient that counts but what the doctor really does. When once the patient realizes that his doctor does walk his talk, the patient's confidence is easily won.

William Osler had this to say to the young medicos of his time: the doctor needs two great qualities of head and heart—imperturbability and aequanimitas. His speech on the occasion of his retirement finally from Johns Hopkins-Aequanimita is a piece worth its weight in gold for all times to come. If the doctor knows communication skills well, diagnosis becomes a pleasure on the bedside. "If you listen to your patient long enough, he/she will tell you what is wrong with him/her," wrote Lord Platt in 1949. Recently, five of his old students, conducted a prospective study using the latest research methods to confirm the truth of Platt's statement in an article in the *BMJ* in 1975 on the role of history-taking and other methods of diagnosis on the bedside!

Confidence builds on the doctor's capacity to *listen* to the patient. Listening is a very difficult art. Every medical student should be trained to master the art of listening. Most of us are good talkers but poor listeners. True listening is to be attentive while the patient pours out his sorrows with appropriate responses as and when needed. Prof Calnan in his very good book *Talking with Patients* elaborates on the art of listening. Henry David Thoreau wrote, "To affect the quality of the day-that is the highest of arts." The art of listening to the patient is the capacity of the doctor to enhance the quality of the patient's day!

Listening to the patient is not confined to simply listing the patients' symptoms, past history, and his social and family history. The crux of the *art of listening* is to understand the patient's fears, his religious, spiritual and social beliefs, his cultural upbringing, and more than all that, his irrational obsessions regarding terminal illnesses. Even if the doctor is a rationalist and thinks that medicine is a pure science, he/she will have to try and understand the irrationality of the patient's thinking to respond to the patient's satisfaction. The medical profession has to understand that the only truth, even in the king of sciences, physics, is the uncertainty principle of Werner Heisenberg and not the Newtonian deterministic predictability laws or Einstein's relativity.

Watenchap is wot whatenchoppen doen science is what the scientists do is the real truth. Science is not *the whole truth*. "Say not," wrote Kahlil Gibran in his book *The Prophet*, "I have found *the truth*", rather say "I have found *a truth."* Science is only a search for the truth. When the chips are down, even the best of rationalists become irrational. Rock Hudson, once President of American Rationalists' Society, went quietly to drink the holy water in Lourdes when he was seriously ill, I am told. People swallow their skepticism when death stares them in the face. If a doctor could understand all this, it is easy to deal with uncertainty on the bedside. Even modern medicine started five thousand years ago as magic, witchcraft, and sorcery on the banks of the river Nile!

The "quiet art of medicine" does stimulate the human immune system, which really heals. Healing is universally possible while curing is rarely an attainable goal in medicine. A healer must have a large heart coupled with a strong and well trained head. Combining humility and wisdom is not impossible, albeit difficult. One should follow the advice given by Jesus to his followers. "Be ye therefore wise like a serpent but harmless like a dove." One of the best books that I could recommend to doctors is *On Doctoring*.

My personal experience since 1956, when I first started seeing patients as a medical student, has been that if I have a genuine interest in the patient's welfare, the patient will have full faith in me. This matters a lot in the final outcome of illness, uncertainty notwithstanding. Faith heals.

FURTHER READING

- Richard Reynolds and John Stone. *On Doctoring*. 1976. (Simon and Schuster, New York).
- Hegde BM. The unrest cure. *J Assoc Physicians of India*. 1997; 47: 730–731.

CHAPTER 44

Need-Based Medical Education

This is an attempt to look at our present day medical education from within, after nearly four decades of my fecund involvement. This is my attempt to think aloud and share my anguish with the reader. Modern medical education in India goes back to the year 1857, when the East India Company started three medical colleges in Madras, Bombay, and Calcutta. The initial syllabus was brought from the London University. It has, of course, changed a bit here and there, but there has never been an attempt to really do some introspection for nearly one-century and a half.

There has never been an attempt to see if our hoary past, with its wonderful medical knowledge, could, at least, be amalgamated with the western thoughts brought from outside, with benefit to the suffering humanity. Most of us inside the system have a holier-than-thou attitude towards anything Indian that has not been certified to be scientific by the West. I think time has come now to think of all that, as the West itself is looking to the East for inspiration in this field with the top heavy, hi-tech western medicine having become prohibitively expensive. A sizeable percentage of the populace in the West is opting out of the system for various reasons, not the least is cost in a fee-for-service system. The London Royal College of Physicians recently brought out a manual, following a symposium on *The Science of Alternative Medicine,* highlighting the positive aspects of the latter and also bringing out a lot of good scientific material in them. It is time now for us to take a fresh look.

Be that as it may, we should also look to see if the present system of teaching and learning are relevant to the scenario obtaining in the world today. There are many questions to be asked and then answered in this area and I shall attempt to do just that. I shall leave the reader to draw his/her own conclusions.

What is Wrong with the Present System?

On the surface everything looks good. Many would want to know that if it was good enough for us why not continue it for the next generation. How good is good? Modern hi-tech medicine, sold all over as very scientific has a very shaky foundation. "*For all its breathtaking progress, modern medicine, like the tower of Pisa, is slightly off balance,*" was the feeling of the outside world, very well represented by Prince Charles, the heir to the British throne, in one of the meetings recently. David Eddy, a former associate professor of cardiovascular surgery at Stanford University, after very extensive research, wrote that 85% of what doctors do is based on very soft data, while only 15% is based on hard unequivocal data. So much for scientific validity.

The recent UNIDO report showed that about 80% of the world's population today does not have the benefit of modern medicine. Many studies have very clearly shown that the most important risk factor for all diseases, from common cold to cancer, is poverty. Poverty and ignorance begin to have their ill effects on the future man right from the first trimester of pregnancy inside his mother's womb and chases him to the tomb! Studies in the West have shown that whereas diseases are plentiful in far-flung villages, surplus of doctors are in the cities and metropolises. This *inverse-care law*, propounded by a family doctor, Tudor Edward Hart, working in a Welsh mining village, speaks volumes about what happens even in third world countries.

The art of medicine, that which makes the patient's day, is not being taught enough in medical schools. Even when passing remarks are made by some teachers about the art of medicine, most of it gets drowned in the sea of awe-inspiring technology. There is a lot we could do in this field, as shown very well by an Oxford professor, David Weatherall, in his book *The Science of Medicine and its Quiet Art*, and by Shervin B Nuland, Stanford professor of clinical surgery, in his book *Wisdom of the Body*. The art of listening, which many times gives the doctor a clue to the diagnosis and management, is forgotten these days in our teaching. Most young men and women in the medical schools feel that it is a waste of time to listen to patients. This has been proved wrong by a very scientific study by a group of professors of medicine in England published in the *BMJ*. Professor Calnan's book *Talking with Patients* brings out the anguish of a thinking teacher at the Hammersmith hospital, London. Too much use of technology and teaching subtleties to undergraduates was shown to be counterproductive in a study by three generations of teachers in the Department of Cardiology at the St. Andrews University, Dundee.

Our replicative evaluation system is another curse for proper learning. The student gets lost in memorizing data for the sake of the examination and thus loses sight of the woods while counting the trees. At the end of the day, what with all the memorizing, the new doctor is not capable of coherently communicating with the sick and their near and dear ones. Bereavement is an integral part of a doctor's life! Very little input is given in this direction for students to cope with it. Memorizing the subject has another dangerous consequence in that the student just before the examination, and if he passes the examination, for ever after deludes himself with the idea that he **knows everything that is to be known.** This feeling of **"knowing"** is suicidal in this field. One should aim at making the student realize genuinely that he **does not know!** That is where curiosity starts and wisdom begins. Our present system breeds **paternalism** in medical care, whereas **partnership should be the better word in dealing with patients.**

I hope, by now, I have been able to convert, at least, a few of the readers to think that there may be room for improvement in this field where, earlier, there was no need to have a re-look at medical education. Another very important reason why medical education has become irrelevant to the present day needs is the craze for trying to do good to the **apparently healthy** in society in the name of **health screening and predicting the unpredictable**. Both these have been highlighted by the BMJ recently. Whereas screening is a very good business proposition for the hospitals and equipment and drug manufacturers, it may not do much good (may even be dangerous) to the population! The reasons are not far to seek.

Predicting the future of any organism in this dynamic universe needs the knowledge of the **total initial state** of the organism, which is impossible today since we have no clue about the genotype of man and his consciousness! In addition, the linear thinking that if one were to change the **initial states from "abnormal" to "normal" there is no guarantee that this change holds good as time evolves.** The very definition of **normality** is fraught with the inherent danger of false positive results. Time evolution in a dynamic system does not follow this rule. Long term studies have shown the futility of this kind of exercise. That doctors have been *predicting the unpredictable* is the judgement of a physicist, professor Firth, put forth in his enlightening article in the *BMJ* in 1991. The same is again highlighted in a good book *Who Has Seen a Blood Sugar?,* by an American professor and diabetologist, Frank Davidoff. Most students do not have an idea of the type of science that is being used in medicine!

What Could be Done to Rectify This?

This could be discussed under three heads, viz., Changes in the content, methods, and evaluation in the medical school to make medical education relevant to the societal needs.

Content and Methodology

The syllabus is already overburdened. It cannot and should not be expanded; instead it could be profitably cut short, without affecting the quality, nay even enhancing the quality of education. Problem-based learning, where the student and the tutor are both curious to learn, would be a better method. More time should be given to the students to think for themselves, in place of all the didactic teaching of facts. Facts keep changing everyday, what with new information pouring in at a phenomenal pace of seven per cent per month. **The correct method of obtaining data from many sources today is to be taught in place of teaching facts.**

The student should be provided with all the opportunities to learn for himself, like a delivering mother who needs care, compassion, love, empathy, and assistance, but the delivering has to be done by the mother herself. Similarly, the student should be given all the above but, the learning has to be done by him. A good teacher, who shows by his example, that learning is not an easy process and that it is a never ending process, would be the ideal example to motivate the student. Longer and prolonged contact between the teacher and the taught, as was done in the ancient Indian *gurukula system,* would be more beneficial.

Didactic lectures could be cut to the bare minimum. Even those should be more of a deliberation on a topic rather than custom-made time bound lecture. The attendance in those lectures must be purely optional to make them more effective. Studies have shown that an unprepared mind absorbs less than five per cent of what is told in a lecture class. That could come down still further if the student has a hostile attitude!

Clinical clerkships must take more of the student's time. There again the ritualistic bedside clinics should give place to collective effort between the teacher and the taught to arrive at the diagnosis and management strategies for every patient under their charge. Then and then only does the student realize the most important lesson in medicine that diagnoses and management are basically full of *uncertainty*. **The only certainty in medicine is uncertainty.** The gray zone in medicine is expanding every day and the student should be aware of that as much as the teacher.

Medical education should be a collective effort at learning between the two parties, the teacher and the taught. The conventional *teaching by humiliation* should give place to learning with pleasure with a footing of equality. On the bedside the student learns by observing the teacher, in all its ramifications, viz., manners, ready wit, compassion, understanding, human dignity, patient leeway, frustrations, anxieties, and what have you. This would give the student the courage to keep learning. The process could be assisted by the thought in the student's mind that even his teacher, under certain special circumstances, lacks total knowledge! To know that the *emperor also could be without his robes* is a very good stimulus to learn.

Specialists vs Generalists

There was a craze for specialization in the West for more than two decades now. There were so many specialties and subspecialties that they have now realized the bad effects of these both on the recipient, the patient, and also on the system. This kind of fragmentation is doomed to fail as per the 1st Law of Thermodynamics! In anything new the Americans lead the way, basically based on the business interest in any field. Medical specialties grew directly proportional to the growth of technology. The result is that technology has become top heavy and hospitals have become prohibitively expensive even for middle class Americans. The trend is reversing now with Universities looking to go back to their old ways.

The University of Minneapolis has started the system of having only three major specialties: general surgery, general medicine and midwifery. They have appointed Professors of general medicine and surgery who oversee the diagnoses and management of most, if not all outpatients. Only when there is a definite indication for any type of intervention does the patient get referred to the particular specialist. Similar trend is coming to the UK also. There are demands for decreasing the cardiac specialty centers even there.

Of course, we Indians believe in the dictum that we have to make the mistakes ourselves before we learn from them. We are not wise enough to learn from other's mistakes. We are where Americans were twenty years ago, starting more and more specialties and corporate hospitals. We would be committing the same mistakes in the future. Even earlier, the UK had a special system where the specialist also had sufficient training in his major branch that he could manage all patients at the first contact.

A large country like India where more than 80% of our patients are spread over the 5,75,000 odd villages, we would have to, per force, have more generalists. In addition, our present day medical training for a graduate is not conducive to send him to a village to manage alone. He would be a fish out of water there, as the ground realities in the community incidence of illnesses is not represented in the teaching hospitals. This is one of the main reasons why doctors do not want to go to the village. New doctors are not comfortable with their clinical abilities sans the hi-tech equipment that they are used to in their medical school hospitals. If every headache patient in the village has to be CAT scanned, the country would go down the drain! But the new graduate would not be comfortable unless he ruled out a very rare small malignant lesion in the brain in a rare patient with headache.

The same holds good for all other patients. Our graduates are good for working as junior doctors in larger corporate hospitals to order all the tests for every one who comes there for the boss to review when he arrives. Left alone in a village he would be helpless. We need to reorient our training.

Evaluation

This is the real pain in the neck for both teachers and students alike. I know of no foolproof method of evaluation. The present system that we follow, which has been followed since the beginning of medical education in India, is far from satisfactory. Even though the best is yet to be thought of, we could try and make it more effective.

The end-of-term, one-time examination should be replaced by continuous on-the-job evaluation. This could be split into teacher evaluation and peer evaluation. The latter could bring out the weaknesses and strengths of a candidate much more candidly. The teacher evaluation should be a long drawn observation in place of the short, anxiety generating, incomplete assessment. The debate about the type of theory examination is a never-ending one. The West went into the multiple choice objective theory tests, only to go back now to the time-tested essay type examination. However, both of them test the memory power of the examinee and not his total ability. In their place a novel creative type of theory examination could be held. The student is posed a real life problem and is given enough time to write a critical answer on the lines of his future work outside. He could consult books if he wants in the examination hall. The question must be such that the student would not be able to copy the whole answer from any book!

No one could be expected to keep all the information in his head these days of explosive knowledge in every field. Even in day-to-day work one will have to consult medical literature when in doubt. The student must be adept at consulting these sources and, if he is found to be good enough, he should be let loose on the gullible public. Parrot repeating a textbook would not stand him in good stead in real life situations. A critical appraisal of the problem should be able to give the candidate the capacity to learn the communication skills in later life also.

Practical and clinical examinations should mimic real life situations. They should aim to assess the candidate's ability to listen to his patient, his compassion and human understanding, his knowledge of the clinical methods of eliciting the signs of disease, his interpersonal relations, his ability to get on with colleagues, his temperament as a doctor, and his mastery of the diagnostic skills and management strategies. To test his ability to communicate could be assessed by asking him to write a discharge letter to the patient's family physician about the patient's clinical status.

Viva-Voce examination is an opportunity to check the student's thinking capacity, instead of once again assessing his memory recall. This could be utilized to find out what kind of a doctor he would make in real life, his interest in furthering his skills and knowledge, his capacity to look at the same thing from different angles and also to fathom his reasoning power.

Examiners should have a check on them. All the markings should be in the *close-marking method,* where each part of the examination (short and long case etc.) should be marked out of ten. Five out of ten or four and six are okay; but if the mark is below 4 out of ten or more than six out of ten the examiner should give in writing the reasons for that particular mark. The positive and negative aspects of the student's abilities should be noted down for the future guidance of the candidate should he fail to make the grade. The examiners' performance should be computerized to assess them as examiners. Erring people should be blacklisted and their names sent to all the examining bodies with valid explanations. They could always be reassessed after the lapse of a particular number of years.

Beyond the Four Walls of the Class Room

Doctoring needs more skills than all that is written above. There are important areas not covered by the conventional teaching methods. One area that needs wider knowledge of human affairs is the capacity of the doctor to handle the only certain thing in life: death. One of the questions asked is *"why"* did a patient get a particular disease or why did he die? These two questions could never be answered in biology. One needs to know a bit of teleology and also philosophy. Positive sciences answer the question "how" or "how much", but not the question "why." One needs special skills of compassion and understanding to manage bereavement and separation.

The bane of modern medicine today is its cost. Every doctor must have an exposure to pharmaco-economics. It is one thing to read a book and write the medicine or order an operation, but the crux of the matter is whether the recipient is able to afford it and if not, what are the alternatives. Many doctors today simply follow the rule of thumb that they have studied in medical school and leave it at that. That leaves the much-harried patient in a worse state. One has to have knowledge of the alternatives available and their scientific validity. Patients have more extensive knowledge of the alternative systems of medicine today than doctors do. One should be aware of the role of complementary systems of medicine in disease control.

The mind of man is known to be the most important part of the whole gamut of health and disease and the modern doctor should be able to unravel the depths of the human mind, with a reasonable knowledge of human psychology, local customs, taboo, fears, anxieties and even superstitious beliefs. An assessment of the patient's surroundings, his worries, his anxieties, his near and dear ones, and his social ties would all have to be taken care of in some special situations. Since the medical course is long and arduous, one could not squeeze all these into the curriculum, but they need be taught all the same and students should be exposed to these situations during their tenure in the medical school. Special guest lectures, workshops, and group discussions could be encouraged.

Knowledge advances by refuting false dogmas. Genuine research demands that doctors keep an open mind on all aspects of their learning and try and get the dogmas demolished to the furthest extent possible. This requires the capacity to keep meticulous records of all dealings with patients sincerely and honestly. Documentation should be taught to students from day one in their routine work as well. Research is not repeating others' work in your laboratory. Clinical medical research is "having a question on the bedside and trying to go as far away from the bed as one could to get an answer."

In this context the new doctor should be trained in the methods of collecting data from the medical literature. The latter could be compared to a jungle full of dead wood. There are occasional rose-woods and teaks inside, but a novice who gets in there without proper guidance may not reach the rose wood, and might even be bitten by a snake or eaten by a tiger. Medical technology and the drug industry would want to twist research data to suit their business interests, and the reader of the medical literature should be trained to pick the wheat from the chaff. This is an ongoing process and one has to keep on learning daily!

In short, medical education is an education for life. The right kind of education would bring out the best in every doctor who becomes patient friendly and would be able to do the most good to most people most of the time. He is ideally **one who knows not, but knows he knows not. May his tribe increase!**

FURTHER READING

- Hegde BM. Need for a change in medical paradigm. *Proc Royal Coll Physi Edin* 1993; 23: 9–12.
- McCormack J, Greenhalgh T. Seeing what you want to see in research- The UPSPD study. *BMJ* 2000; 320: 1720–1723
- Rang M. The Ulysses Syndrome, *Can Med Assn J* 1972; 106: 122–123.
- Brody, Jane and Denise Grady, *The New York Times Guide to Alternative Health*. New York: New York Times Co., 2001. 203–244.
- Angell M. Is academic medicine for sale? *N Engl J Med* 2000; 342: 1516-8
- Clinton B. Science in the 21st Century, *Science* 1997; 276: 1951.
- Charles Townes. Of lasers and Prayers. *Science* 1997; 277: 891.

CHAPTER 45

Health Care Delivery in India Today

The thinking that doctors and hospitals are needed to keep the society healthy is plain rubbish.

—*MacFarlane Burnett*

The quotation from Burnett was necessary to drive home the point that health care delivery is not synonymous with, and has very little to do with, illnesses and the quick-fix "cures" that are sold in the media by the establishment, for every conceivable disease. Health is the holistic aspect of man's creative existence on this planet. Man is born to contribute his mite to society. To do that he must have all the following—physical, mental, social and spiritual wellbeing. Mere absence of bodily illnesses does not necessarily make a man healthy in the true sense. Even people with advanced incurable diseases are, at times, more creative and "healthy" than most of us. The shining example would be the well-known physicist, Stephen Hawkins, who cannot even lift a little finger of his hands because of a peculiar disease, amyotrophic lateral sclerosis, has possibly done more than any of his peers for furthering the cause of theoretic physics. Spiritual health deals with man's relation with nature and teaches him the significance of his inter-dependence in this universe.

The Indian scenario in health care is unique. While the standards of health care, measured by infant mortality and maternal deaths, reach European standards in Kerala and the West Coast, it is worse than sub-Saharan Africa in most parts of Bihar and eastern Uttar Pradesh. One cannot possibly apply one single yardstick for the whole of India. The methods should be need-based to suit the geographic disparity. Our production rate in most places is outstripped by our reproduction rate. We add every year an extra population equivalent to that of the continent of Australia. In addition, the alcohol and the tobacco lobby add a huge burden of illnesses to our already depleted health delivery machinery. Their advertisements seem to reach our masses better than all our slipshod efforts at health education. It is shocking to know that even today more than half of our children have only less than 50% haemoglobin in their blood. This is due to the lack of toilet facilities in villages and even in city slums, leading to very heavy hookworm load. To just give one example, in the whole state of Bihar only less than 5% of the population has sanitary facilities!

The real India, which lives in more than 5, 75, 000 villages, needs the following simple measures to be kept healthy:

- Clean drinking water, which avoids almost 80% of gut diseases.
- Avoidance of their food being contaminated by human and/or animal excreta.
- Three square meals a day.
- Economic empowerment to avoid the greatest stress in life, i.e.,: not knowing where the next meal comes from! Poverty is the mother of all illnesses.
- Avoiding cooking smoke (worse than tobacco smoke) from getting into the house. The latter could be very dangerous for the lungs of children below five years of age.
- Keep people properly informed about the immunization facilities for their children. This should be done very carefully lest drug companies should misuse this to sell some dubious vaccines to school children by influencing the teachers and parents.
- Trained health workers, selected from among able bodied, high school educated boys and girls, belonging to the village, to be trained for a period of six months to a year to identify illnesses needing hospitalization and emergency treatment. Such patients could be sent directly to the nearest hospital. These boys and girls could also administer innocuous drugs for the common illness syndromes, which are more common than we think they are.
- They could also be trained to help with immunization and nutritional needs of the pregnant mothers.
- There are a few drugs that have no power to kill someone even if given in horse doses by mistake. The quacks use a lot more drugs with impunity and most of them are very successful practitioners anyway, having been legally allowed to do so! The present day primary health centers are but a menace if one seriously thinks about their economics and their role in keeping the health of the villagers and looking after the sick.

What Doctors Don't Get to Study in Medical School

The health care delivery that the media sells daily is, in effect, medical care delivery—delivery of the hi-tech western medical quick fixes to a gullible public. Please make a clear distinction between the two lest you should mistake one for the other. While genuine health care delivery is what we should be doing, we waste the taxpayers' money on illusory medical care instead, in the most illogical way! Our politicians want the five-star hospital culture in their areas! The latter is slowly dying in the West.

How did this mistake in thinking come about that hospitals would be the be-all and end-all of health care? Medical education was based on the filtered lot of patients who reach the teaching hospitals. One of the studies in Canada in this direction recently showed that if one thousand people fell sick in a society only one man eventually landed up in a teaching hospital. Consequently, the student does not get to see the real spectrum of diseases in society and gets a distorted picture of the latter. One example would suffice.

Out of thousand people getting some sort of a pain or ache in the chest region, one man would have serious coronary artery disease. The medical student and his teachers in the five-star set-up get to see only that filtered one person and repeatedly the student gets reinforced with the mistaken notion that every chest pain patient suffers from coronary artery disease and needs investigations! The rest of the nine hundred and ninety nine people, if they happen to see these doctors, suffer from over-investigation with all its bad effects on their health and purse, commonly labeled as Ulysses syndrome.

The few doctors who took to public health medicine did very little to make the medical world realize the gravity of the situation. Whereas the marginal fall in mortality and morbidity claimed in the USA in the last two decades was mainly (54%) due to the change of mode of living and sanitation with the modern vaccinations, only a small fraction of the decrease (only 3.4%) was due to all the hi-tech stuff that we go to town with. Despite that, only urative doctors, the *"star performers"* among them, led by the surgeons doing heroic surgeries (patient as the hero, though) get the limelight and television cover. The poor public health personnel that are responsible for the major changes do not get to be seen or heard.

The society, therefore, gives all the credit to curative quick-fix methods, most of which are not even audited. That is how the medi-business lobby wants to sell their wares and technologies. In retrospect, some of the commonly used technologies have been found to be doing more harm than good when audited. The only disease man was able to conquer, smallpox, was eradicated with public health measures and not using any hi-tech stuff.

There was a shocking revelation that in the year 1998 there were an estimated 100,000 deaths in USA due only to medical mistakes. In a scary report (IOM report) in 2000 it was revealed that USA's health care is the worst among the 14 industrialised countries although USA ranks among the best in life style changes that have taken place in the west in the last half a century! The report also revealed that hospitals and doctors' interventions were the third important cause of death in that country followed by the fourth cause being Adverse Drug Reactions (ADRs). If that were so, one could imagine the scenario in other less developed countries that try and ape the USA! Newer drugs and technologies that were not audited could have contributed a major share to those deaths. Only one example is enough to gauze the gravity of the situation. One of the commonly used technologies in the intensive care set up, the Swan-Ganz catheter, was estimated to have caused havoc with patients' lives! Many drugs give rise to iatrogenic (doctor induced) diseases.

Some drugs are necessary evils, but many of the ill-effects could be avoided by more judicious use of the drugs. Parsimonious use of painkillers and antibiotics could reduce harm substantially. While the above two groups of drugs could be life saving in rare situations, they are mostly used unnecessarily resulting in more harm both at the time of use and sometimes at a future date. Use of antibiotics in common viral upper respiratory tract infections in small children is now known to be one of the triggers for asthma in later life.

Another area needing urgent audit is the vast area of preventive screening of the apparently healthy population with the promise of doing good and to detect diseases in their incipient stage for better control and early cure. The truth is otherwise. Most of the screening procedures, audited so far, have shown that they do more harm than good. Time evolution does not depend on partial knowledge of man at any given time; it needs total initial knowledge. The latter in our present wisdom is not possible since we cannot measure man's mind (consciousness) that forms about 40% of him. Neither could we correctly assess the role of the genes in our present knowledge. The genome map has belied our hope that we would be able to detect a gene fault for every human ill and then be able to set it right. We have about twice as many genes as the round worm and the touted genetic engineering, has come to naught in most disease states except a few. Doctors have been predicting the unpredictable in human illnesses.

The fault partly lies in the modern medical education. While the pattern of illnesses in the community is not represented in the hospital population where teaching goes on, future doctors get a distorted vision of the real life situations. Some of them unlearn what they learnt at medical school to relearn the real medicine in the community, but the percentage of the latter is very small indeed. Most practise what they had learnt at school. We need to reorient our medical education to be mainly community based, to rectify this fault.

With this background the recent news about the doctors' strike in Israel last year (March and April 2000) having resulted in a remarkable fall in mortality and morbidity, does not come as a surprise. Similar experiences had been reported in smaller communities in the past in Canada and Los Angeles County. In fact, in one of them it was the morticians that brokered peace between the doctors and their employers. Doctors' strike must have hit the morticians' business very badly.

That said, I must hasten to add that good doctoring is a must for society and could do a lot for the suffering humanity. Problem comes only when we do not let the "well" alone! Medical establishment could definitely avert many serious emergencies with timely intervention, all suffering could be very effectively controlled by modern methods and a good doctor could console even dying patients and their relatives, even in those situations where death becomes inevitable. A kind-hearted doctor could never be dispensed with in society even when man goes to live on the moon.

The basic problem with health care delivery is the *Inverse Care Law* that operates in this field. While most illnesses affect the poor and the deprived in far off villages and inaccessible areas, most of the doctors and the star-performers crowd round large metropolitan cities even in the developed West. Health education of the masses is absent in areas of poverty and is totally distorted in those places with easy access to information. Most drug companies and/or technology manufacturers doctor health-related lay publications. A recent study in America showed that even medical education there is run by the money from the two above-mentioned sources! Research is no respecter of good practices either. If you look the gift horse in the mouth, you would get to see most researchers to be in the pay roll of the med-business.

The last, but the most important, reason for all the mess that we are in, is the use of wrong methods and mathematics in medical research. While the human body is a dynamic structure, we use linear mathematical rules. This is the reason why we have been missing the benefits that accrue from yoga, mediation, prayer and many other mundane methods in health delivery. Studies now reveal that the human mind is at the root of all human ills. It is not what one eats that kills, but it is what eats one (his negative thoughts) that kills him much more than the food. Most killer diseases originate in the mind from negative thoughts like hatred, greed, jealousy and anger.

In conclusion, it is better that a developing country like India does not follow the footsteps of USA but, follow the path best suited for its special needs. About ten per cent of the illnesses need the hi-tech modern methods for treatment; most of them are in the emergency stage. The majority of the rest of the patients could be helped by other complementary systems of medicine. Ayurveda, the ancient Indian system of medicine, is considered to be the mother of all other systems, including modern medicine. We could make the best use of the latter for health care delivery. Proper training is a pre-requisite for implementation of these methods. The needs of the poor, mentioned in the beginning, should get top priority. I hope we will one day be able to achieve success with this approach.

FURTHER READING

- Hegde BM. The unrest cure. *J Assoc Physi India.* 1997; 47: 730–731.
- Angell M. Is academic medicine for sale? *N Engl J Med* 2000; 342: 1516-8.
- Editorial. Drug Company influence on medical education in USA. *Lancet* 2000; 356: 781–83.
- Firth WJ. Chaos-Predicting the unpredictable. *BMJ* 1991; 303: 1565–1568.
- Andersson OK, Almgren T, Persson B et al. Survival in treated hypertension: follow up after two decades. *BMJ* 1998; 317: 167–171.
- Stewart-Brown S, Farmer A. Screening could seriously damage your health. *BMJ* 1997; 314:533.
- Pickering WG. Does medical treatment mean patient benefit? *Lancet* 1996;347: 379–80.
- Campbell EG, Louis KS, Blumenthal D. looking a gift horse in the mouth. *JAMA* 1999; 279: 995–999.
- Rang M. The Ulysses Syndrome, *Can Med Assn J* 1972; 106: 122–123.
- Starfield B. Is US medicine the best in the world? *JAMA* 2000; 284: 483–485.

CHAPTER 46

Eye of the Beholder

I once glanced through an editorial in *The Lancet* entitled *Could Epidemiologists Cause Epidemics?* Stimulating title indeed! As I read on, I could feel my thoughts beautifully verbalized in the editorial. Story goes that two young epidemiologists predicted an epidemic of influenza in their country in one of their "scientific" studies. Lo and behold, the incidence of influenza did reach epidemic proportions very soon and their predictions were claimed to be a true warning and were hailed as a milestone study in the media. It is only after serious efforts to reevaluate the epidemic data that the truth came out.

While the fear of the epidemic ran through the medical profession and also the populace, there was more labeling. Every fever in the intensive therapy unit became an influenza attack and people rushed to the hospitals with even questionable rise in body temperature. Concurrently, the incidence of pneumonia in the intensive therapy units went down proportionately. **The final conclusion of the second study was that the apparent increase of influenza was not an absolute increase, but a spurious labeling error.**

Similar serious studies have debunked the epidemiologists' predictions of epidemics of coronary artery disease in this century. The story repeats here as well. Stehaben's studies, published in *The Lancet,* have unequivocally shown that the apparent rise in coronary disease was due to increased labelling. Every sudden death was labeled as a myocardial infarction. Large number of cardiomyopathies due to alcohol did result in sudden electric death, but the label of myocardial infarction was applied there as well. The story goes on and on. The *Shopping Plaza* blood pressure check ups threw up an epidemic of hypertension in America and sent sick-absenteeism skyrocketing. Recent studies of diabetes are trying to do the same. They are predicting a big epidemic of diabetes in the next century.

While all this makes good business sense for the *fix-it* trade, it is a sad commentary on the truth in science. It is very logical that any disease-statistics applied to the normal healthy population should result in large false positives. While the debate about screening healthy populations to predict the future may only be an academic discussion, the resulting treatment strategies could harm people in many ways. A revolutionary study of **quality of life** done in insulin-treated diabetics clearly showed that the real relief came only to those patients **who were symptomatic before treatment. For those asymptomatic diabetics there was, if anything, worsening of the quality of life with treatment.** The million-dollar question, however, was did this reduce long-term consequences? The question could not be answered by this short-term study. **But the trend in the study showed that it did not reduce long-term consequences.**

It is time-honoured logic that when a patient goes to the doctor with symptoms, it is the duty of the doctor to do his best for the patient's suffering, even if the knowledge in that field, at that point in time, might not be unequivocally in favor of the line of management. We are on a very wet wicket when it comes to trying to fix things for the apparently healthy population, in the fond hope of preventing future suffering.

Let me remind the reader of the famous saying of a great medical brain, Sir William Osler: **"patient doing well do not interfere!"** There is an editorial in the *British Medical Journal* warning doctors that **screening could seriously damage your health!** The unhealthy life style of this century, not seen in the centuries gone by, could, of course, be changed for the better. This specially applies to our food habits at the present time, as well as the fatal smoking and alcohol habits. Sedentary living is another of our enemies. Monetary economy with its attendant greed and hatred could cut the very roots of good health!

Predictions of the future rarely come true even in other scientific fields, including the king of sciences, physics. Edward Lorenz, after bagging the Nobel for his innovative ideas of weather predictions, realized that weather predictions rarely came true! He, then, propounded the **butterfly effect.** Said he: "after feeding all the data in the traffic rules of air currents into the super computer, if a butterfly were to move its wings in Beijing, there could be storms in New York after a month!" This happens in all the dynamic systems. **"Doctors have been predicting the unpredictable,"** wrote Professor Firth in his mile stone paper in the *British Medical Journal*.

In any dynamic system, like the human body, the future depends on the total initial knowledge of the organism. To predict the future of man one should know his phenotype (that is what our screening procedures do), his genotype, and his consciousness. We do not have any inkling into the latter two major aspects of human existence now. Even if we know any deviation in the phenotype, there is no truth in predicting that **correcting the initial deviation in the body would hold good as time evolves to the benefit of the person.** It could even go against him! We have been seeing this time and again in blood pressure screening, diabetes screening, and even cancer surveys. Truth cannot be hidden for all times, although falsehood and mystery would drag millions by the nose at a given time.

"Man seeth what he wisheth" is an old adage. Man sees what he knows, right! Even the eye of the beholder could not tell him the real truth unless he examines the object carefully. This is the real meaning of science with its Sanskrit etymological root, **skei**, meaning just the same (cut into what you see). This reminds me of the famous **Schrödinger's cat.** In the early part of this century when quantum physics upset the apple cart of Einstein's theory of relativity, first by his own student, Werner Heisenberg, with his **uncertainty principle,** and later by Erwin Schrödinger, an Austrian physicist, Einstein must have been very much hurt. His elephantine ego did not make him understand both these great brains. The very fact that he ruled that **"nothing could move faster than light"** showed his closed mind and arrogance. All quantum particles could move much faster than light! He claimed that **"if Schrödinger's quantum physics is to be believed, this world would look crazy, but one would have to assess how crazy!"**

At the quantum level (sub-atomic level) whether we exist or not depend on someone observing us, the eye of the beholder. Schrödinger's imagination threw up his cat in a sealed box. The cat lived there in the company of a triggering device and a decaying atom. The atom would decay in an hour's time and trigger the alarm. One would know if the cat were alive or dead only after opening the box and looking. Although Schrödinger's cat provoked much discussion and debate in the world, a recent attempt by physicists to prove the theory wrong did not bear fruit. They tried to pass a mouse in front of the cat inside the box, but that did not make the cat mew, thereby proving that the question of life and death of the cat depended solely on seeing the cat after opening the box by the observer.

Medical scientists will have to learn a lot from quantum physics, including its elucidation of human consciousness as a sub-atomic concept. Mind could not be confined either to the brain or the heart as was done by our modern medical forefathers. The brain has only about hundred billion cells, but even a grain of salt has more than ten billion atoms. Consequently, brain cells could not be the seat of the mind. In the latter event even a grain of salt could not have been understood by the human mind! Mind and matter are two things that have been ignored by us for a long time with disastrous consequences for our patients.

Both in the Indian system of Ayurveda and, even, in modern medicine there have been attempts to lay stress on the role of the mind in disease. William Harvey so graphically described the role of the mind in disease when he wrote in 1648 AD: *"when in anger the pupils contract, in infamy and shame the cheeks blush, in lust does the member get distended and erected in no time!"* Indian science of Ayurveda had clearly stated that health depends on a happy mind to a very great extent:

Prasanna aathma indriya manah swastha ithyabhideeyathe.
(Happiness of the soul, senses, and the mind keep you healthy)

We should spend more time and energy in trying to do most good to most people most of the time, by trying to alleviate suffering. Hippocrates did warn us about our responsibilities when he said: **"Cure rarely, comfort mostly, but console always."** This is true even today! In addition, we have made modern medicine so expensive, what with all our the screenings and gadgetry, that more than 62% of upper middle class Americans find it difficult to have health insurance. "In a fee-for-service system, cardiac procedures generated billions of dollars each year. A high volume of procedures brought prestige and financial rewards to hospitals, physicians, and the vendors of medical equipment." This was the opinion expressed by an American professor of cardiology in a recent editorial in the *New England Journal of Medicine.* A recent UNIDO report showed that about 80% of the world's population is still not aware of modern medicine. Recent scientific studies published by the *Royal College of Physicians of London* have revealed that many of the complementary systems of medicine could be scientific and, do have a role to play in health care delivery.

Let us be pragmatic in our approach to health care, taking a holistic view of health and disease, to bring succor to the suffering. We should not waste our energy and money in claiming to lessen the burden of illness by *catching diseases young,* a myth at this point in time. Let epidemiologists be more careful in predicting the unpredictable future. We still have millions of people in the world that need help for their suffering. If we look out for anything in particular with zeal, we, probably, get to see it more often. Consequently we feel like intervening, where angels fear to tread! This reminds me of what Mark Twain once wrote:

For a man with a hammer in the hand and wanting to use it badly, everything here looks like a nail needing hammering!

FURTHER READING

- Editorial: Do epidemiologists cause epidemics? *Lancet* 1993;341:993–94.
- Stehbens WE. An appraisal of epidemic rise of coronary heart disease and its decline. *Lancet* 1987;I:606–611
- Ramachandran A. The Scenario is not sweet. *The Hindu*, 30th Dec, 1998.
- Goddijn PPM, Bilo HJG, Feskens EJM et al. Longitudinal study on glycaemic control and quality of life in patients with Type II diabetes. *Diabetic Med*. 1993;16:23–30.
- Stewart-Brown S, Farmer A. Screening could seriously damage your health. *BMJ* 1997;314: 533.
- Ornish D, Scherwitz LW, Billings JH. et al. Intensive life-style changes for reversal of coronary heart disease. *JAMA* 1998; 280; 2001–2008.
- Firth WJ: Chaos-Predicting the Unpredictable. *BMJ* 1991; 303: 1565–1568.
- Krumholz HM: Cardiac procedures, outcomes, and accountability. *N Engl J Med* 1997; 336: 1522–23.
- Meade T: *Science-based complementary medicine*. Ed. Royal College of Physicians London, 1999.

CHAPTER 47

Need for a Paradigm Shift in Medical Philosophy

The art of progress is to preserve order amid change, and to preserve change amid order.

—*Alfred North Whitehead*

"Time has come," the Walrus said, "to talk of many things—cabbages and kings..." Time, really, has come to talk of an urgent need for a paradigm shift in the medical establishment's thinking and philosophy, if there is one in place already. Walrus, of course, had his next meal in mind when he was saying this to the crabs, but the present dialogue has anything but altruism as its inspiration!

The present thinking and teaching in medicine is that doctors are trained to cure illnesses, as also to prevent diseases by detecting them in their early asymptomatic stage and then try to correct the presumed "abnormalities", with the assistance of drugs and technology that we have at our command. In the bargain if one could make money that much better. More money one makes the merrier. Doctoring has never been taught as a discipline to keep the health of the public. Sadly, health as a concept has not been fully understood in the modern medical thinking, as health can not be a reductionist concept. **Health needs the preservation of physical, psychological, emotional, spiritual, social, economic, and altruistic wellbeing. Health, therefore, is holistic, could never be a reductionist concept.**

The other major premise in modern medicine is the **reductionist science** that forms its base. This science makes it easy for us to divide the human body into smaller and smaller bits—organs, cells, molecules, chromosomes and genes—and then try to find out the defects in them to be fixed. These quick-fix solutions have eventually led to the belief that setting the genes right would set the man right. Consequently, it strengthens the belief that stem cell research would solve most, if not all, problems of mankind. I wish it were true. **The cloning experiment itself has not been successful so far. Even the genetically modified gene therapy in the first three children has resulted in unexpected cancers in those children**! Genetically modified drugs generally have met with similar fate.

Many of the surgical and other interventions have never been audited before being let loose on the gullible public. Most of them have fallen by the wayside after the ravages caused by them were brought to notice. Many an intervention has been abandoned. The story of the multitude of drugs-derived again by studying their molecules, either chemical or herbal, have then been studied by the double blind controlled studies, touted as the most scientific method of drug evaluation. The truth, however, is that the medical profession has been blind to the after effects of these double blind studies. In addition, **no drug to date** has been studied in combination with other drugs in a single patient at one time. In real life that is the rule rather than an exception. All the controlled studies are done on a single drug in ideal experimental set ups that are far removed from the ground realities of the real life situations in patient care on an individual basis. This is not true science but statistical science only.

Statistics, used liberally in those studies, have a limited role in that they probably work in large cohorts of men and women, the higher the number the better, but they do not seem to have any bearing on the individual patients that doctors are called upon to treat in their practice. Extrapolating such statistical significance to patient care could have limited role. Human beings could never be put into watertight compartments. Two human beings are never alike. Even the uniovular twins have their genetic differences and, if brought up separately, have many other differences in their physiology. How, then, could we compare two age, sex and body mass index matched groups as identical for controlled studies? Most, if not all, controlled studies have recorded their observations, even those mismatched cohorts, for not more than a maximum of five years. But those drugs are used in practice for many, many years and, in some instances, for the rest of patient's life. Many of those drugs, on retrospective audits, have given rise to serious side effects. Almost every fourth patient on prescription drugs on long term basis has had serious side effects. The individuals taking those drugs on long-term basis do feel that their life is prolonged but have met their maker earlier than scheduled! Adverse Drug Reactions have been the fourth most important cause of death in the USA.

If one tries to overstand the medical scenario from outside the compound wall of secrecy that doctors have built around themselves, one would soon realize that doctors probably have not done enough to preserve health of the public. In the bargain they have, unwittingly, contributed to higher intervention rates in society, resulting in unwanted death and disability as the inevitable fall out of those interventions. **Health preservation requires a strong political will in any country**. The basic needs to preserve health are *clean drinking water*, *empowerment of the public with knowledge and money, providing them with three square meals a day and a roof on their heads*. It is also necessary to give *basic sanitary facilities* like *toilets in every house and avoid deadly cooking smoke* from coming into the house in villages.

Poverty is not only the mother and the womb of all ills, it is also a double-edged sword in that it makes the victim poorer when he/she is ill, robbing him/her of the capacity to work and earn. Of course, one sees the *inverse care law* working in these areas as well. Whereas there are surfeit of doctors in metropolitan cities where they are not needed that much, there are very few in the remote villages where their need is greatest. So be it. A recent audit did show that more doctors in a place do not make the public healthier. Israeli cities did have a remarkable fall in death rate when doctors went on strike for three months in the year 2000, only to come back to the previous level when doctors returned to work!

The new paradigm looks at the human body as a whole, working in tune with nature. The cheapest and the safest way to remain healthy are to preserve the wellness that man is heir to right from birth. Minimum intervention, when inevitable, should be the motto. Ayurveda, the great Indian medical wisdom of yore, has the ideal prescription for preserving health.

Swasthashya swastha rakshitham
(Keep the well healthy)

This should be the new paradigm not only to keep people healthy as long as they live, but also to save them from the ravages of the screening-intervention-iatrogenesis loop. When one gets into that loop it is impossible to come out of that. Man, a well man, becomes a patient the minute he sees a doctor. He, rarely ever, if ever, becomes a well man again! In the modern medical paradigm *a well man is one who has not been completely and properly evaluated. This has become an economic necessity in medicine, as the initial cost of having a set up for screening and intervention is prohibitively expensive.* Recently an American hospital, Tenet Hospital in Reading in Northern California, was closed as the FBI found them intervening most of the time even without indications. The cardiac interventions top the list since they are the biggest money spinners, netting billions of dollars in cash as also prestige to hospitals, doctors and instrument vendors.

Heavy exercise could be detrimental in the long run. Healthy food, preferably vegetarian, taken in moderation, with four helpings of fresh fruit daily would ensure good health. Adequate water intake is a must. **Alcohol and tobacco should be kept as far away as possible. The myth that small quantities of alcohol, especially wine, would promote health is a fraud on the public. Repeated good studies, both prospective and retrospective, have shown NO BENEFIT from alcohol as far as health is concerned.**

The key element in the new paradigm is the important role played by the human mind in human health. Diseases originate in the mind. Destructive emotions and negative thoughts like anger, jealousy, pride, hatred, and depression are the main killers. The educational system should change to inculcate positive thoughts of love, compassion, camaraderie, co-operation, and altruism early in life. Latest scientific findings show that these positive and negative emotions stimulate different parts of the human brain.

Mind does not just reside in the brain, though. Even creatures, which do not have brains, do have emotions. Single cell amoeba knows where to get its food as also to move in that direction. Ants and termites do not have brains. They are blind as well. They still have a collective consciousness that makes them do wonders like building multi-storied anthills. Every cell in the human body has the mind, the consciousness, which in turn is a part of the Universal consciousness. Memory "T" cell in different organs is a good example.

The idea of curing diseases in the present thinking is anything but impossible. The word "*cure*" connotes the capacity to bring back to the original level. Nothing in the human body could be made normal again even after a minor illness, like common cold. Many of the cells in the nasal mucous membrane in common cold are destroyed permanently. The new paradigm talks of healing. **Healing** is pregnant with meaning. The concept tries to make a "whole" of the sick human being. This is possible. The present teaching seems to have forgotten the advice given by Hippocrates, the father of modern medicine: **"to cure rarely, comfort mostly, but console always."** Healing, though, requires a physician who is compassionate and understanding. He should be able to talk with patients and not talk to patients. He should never try to make money in the sick room. Medical education should aim at preserving the health of the public and not at trying to confine himself to making a sophisticated diagnosis and intervening at any cost for monetary gains.

The latest craze in this direction is the introduction of the *whole body scanner* in America. The company is trying to sell those scanners with a vengeance. These machines are supposed to allay anxiety. In reality, they only add anxiety to the whole society since no one will come out of those without something somewhere falling outside the defined "normality." In fact, allaying anxiety is the main goal of the medical establishment—patient anxiety of death and disability and the doctor anxiety of having done enough or not for the patient. Whole body scanner of the conventional school of thought is not the answer. In the new paradigm a **placebo** doctor is the answer to the whole riddle. Long live doctoring for the good of mankind.

> There is a time for departure even when there's no certain place to go.
>
> —*Tennessee Williams*

Further Reading

- Starfield B. Is US Medicine the best in the world? *JAMA* 2000; 284: 483–485.
- Hegde BM. Need for a change in medical paradigm. *Proc Royal Coll Physi Edinb.* 1993; 23: 9–12.
- Krumholz HM. Cardiac Procedures, outcomes, and accountability. *N Engl J Med* 1997; 336; 1522–23
- Stewart-Brown S, Farmer A. Screening could seriously damage your health. *BMJ* 1997; 314: 533.
- Pickering WG. Does medical treatment mean patient benefit? *Lancet* 1996;347: 379–80.

CHAPTER 48

Modern Medicine and Ancient Indian Wisdom

Modern medicine started five thousand years ago on the banks of the river Nile as magic, sorcery, witchcraft, and mumbo-jumbo. It has developed over the years into what is now called scientific modern medicine. But even to this day modern medicine has remained essentially an art based on science.

Unfortunately, it has not been able to fulfill two of its avowed objectives. More than 80% of the world population, a good 4.6 billion people, even today does not seem to be in touch with it; 57% of Britons in a survey expressed their desire to avoid it, if possible; while 62% of upper middle class Americans find it difficult to afford health insurance. The insurance premia, based on star performers' fees, in a fee-for-service system, are prohibitively high.

Prince Charles, the heir to the British throne, was not far off the mark when he remarked some time ago that "modern medicine, for all its breathtaking advances, is slightly off balance like the Tower of Pisa."

The desire of young medicos, both in the UK and the USA, to acquire a working knowledge of other systems of medicine, better called complementary medicine, and the public demand for the latter, resulted in the London College of Physicians organizing a symposium on the Science of Complementary Medicine, a couple of years ago. The French Govt. seems to have saved lots of unnecessary expenditure on health care after they opened a one hundred bed Chinese medicine hospital in Paris.

While it is true that modern hi-tech medicine is very essential for all types of emergency care, ranging from accidents to heart attacks, chronic degenerative diseases still elude any solution. With all the so-called hi-tech, that has been aptly described as middle level technology by Lewis Thomas in his celebrated book, *The Lives of a Cell*, we have been able to eradicate only one disease, small pox. This was possible, not through any of the hi-tech methods, but by simple vaccination.

Ancient Indian wisdom in medicine, like in many other fields of human endeavour, comes from the time honoured Vedic Wisdom. The appendices of the Vedas, the upaangaas, deal with all aspects of human life. The leading among them is Ayurveda, the science of life. This deals with the whole gamut of human health and illnesses. Although Max Muller assessed the age of the Vedas to be around 2500–3000 years, there is unequivocal data to show that they are at least 10000–15000 years old, if not older. In one sense, they have no beginning.

It is a pity that this most ancient system was the only one being ignored in the recent Royal College symposium. There are evidences to show that even some of the Chinese systems, like acupuncture and Qi gong, have emanated from Indian Vedic wisdom, and then migrated with Buddhism to China. Wisdom is not confined to any race, region, time or for that matter, even individuals.

An attempt is made to show in this paper some of the milestones in medicine that show so much similarity between ancient Indian wisdom and modern scientific medicine. I have to, per force, confine myself to only a few of them for the purview of this paper.

In his classic book *India in Greece*, written in 1852, E Pococke gives detailed evidence to show how western civilization came to Greece from Sumeria, and came to Sumeria from India thousands of years earlier. There was large-scale migration of Indian scholars to Greece along with their texts. This ancient classic, India in Greece, is chronicled by Dr Laxmikantham, professor of Mathematics at the Florida Institute of Technology, in his recent book, *The Origin of Human Past*.

In fact, it was Albert Einstein who said: "We owe a debt of gratitude to the Indians, for they taught us how to count, without which no scientific discovery was ever possible."

The Vedic scriptures, including Ayurveda, have always been concerned with the whole of humanity and not just Indians. It does not profess religion in the conventional sense. It has no religious organization or authority and does not deal with **Saguna Brahman**, God with a form. Vedas proclaimed "Vasudhai eva kutumbikam" —the whole world is but one large family.

It was the French astronomer, Bailley, who verified the claims of the ancient Indian astronomers that the most ancient of all systems compared to the Egyptians, Greeks, Romans, and even Jews was the Indian wisdom and all the others derived their conclusions from Indian sources, although most western scholars wanted to debunk Bailley's theories. One such very influential scholar was Reverend Burgess, who in 1860 AD tried in vain, to prove that India was not the cradle of language, mythology, arts, sciences, and religion.

The science of Ayurveda tries to explain how one should look after his body in terms of diet and lifestyle. It talks about medicines only in rare circumstances. It emphasizes the importance of the study of human anatomy and physiology as the basis of all further studies with the help of a dead body; carefully studying every part of the body to understand its functions. It also emphasizes the need for continuous research and study during the doctor's lifetime to keep abreast of new discoveries and theories.

Ayurvedic surgery, led by Shusruta, included amputations, grafting, setting fractures, removal of the foetus, removal of bladder stones, and the eternally famous rhinoplasty that he is known for even to this day. His treatise contained a total of 127 instruments; some of which look very modern, even by today's standards! Brain surgery, drug dynamics, counteracting the effects of poisonous gases and even the present-day Caesarian sections have all been graphically described.

There is now ample evidence to show that "Hippocrates borrowed his materia medica from Ayurvedic sources." The Chinese system of acupuncture, which describes the point locations on the body, the marmas, was described in detail in Ayurveda much earlier. A recent publication from the former USSR Library of the Academy of Sciences, Leningrad, shows how the art of acupuncture originated in India and moved to China. A Chinese Sanskrit scholar, Itszin, who visited India in 637 AD to study at the University of Nalanda, wrote: "the inhabitants of India are imparting proper medical knowledge to the Chinese people in the complete art of treatment by pricking, cauterization and also the study of the pulse." All these show how ancient the Indian system of medicine is.

In modern medicine there are increasing appeals for a unified holistic approach to integrate the somatic and the psychological features of the patient with his or her medical disorder. **However, we still frequently find a disturbing polarization of natural science oriented vs psycho social science oriented medicine.** This division has its roots in the traditional Cartesian division of res cogitans (thinking substance) and res extensa (extended or corporeal substance)—the dualism of subject and object, mind and body. Psychosomatic problems have received much medical attention in the recent times, especially in the neurosciences. This distinction does not exist in Ayurveda.

If only modern medicine could incorporate the knowledge of modern quantum physics more effectively, we could achieve a quantum jump in our effort to overcome the polarization and conflicts caused by dualistic thinking. The traditional thinking in medicine up until now has been based predominantly on the natural sciences of the classical rather than of modern physics, which is based mainly on quantum theory.

If analysis of the human body continues beyond the level of cells, molecules, and atoms to the level of subatomic structures or elementary particles, the old concepts will no longer hold good. Modern physics assumed that elementary particles can no longer be understood as corporeal structures in the sense of the Cartesian res extensa and res cogitans and can only be described without contradictions as mathematical structures. The physicist Heisenberg even referred to these mathematical structures as being closely related to Plato's forms. Thus, in modern natural sciences, the Cartesian concept of res extensa and res cogitans can no longer be consistently maintained.

Medicine must respond to new developments in its natural scientific base and reshape its own position with regard to them. The traditional strict division between psyche and soma must be overcome and the unified holistic approach to the patient should be encouraged.

The history of medical thought in the West has been a succession of errors in the ascending road of progress. Primitive medical concepts and practices began with the first man on earth and have not entirely disappeared today. 99% of man's time on earth—in excess of one million years—ended at about 8000 BC and has been called the Paleolithic period. Surgery of the primitive people had an astonishing degree of technical efficiency. The most ancient instruments were but sharpened stones. Trephining of the skull was carried out among Neolithic people to remove splinters and fragments of fractured skull, for magical purposes to relieve evil spirits etc. Thus mystic faith and empiric experience based upon seeing and believing were the first attitudes adopted by the primitive physician.

What Doctors Don't Get to Study in Medical School

We shall now look at some milestones in the medical world.

Vaccination against Small Pox

Lewis Thomas, former President of the Sloane Kettering Cancer Institute, claims that the highest technology in medicine is the complete understanding of any disease to be able to eradicate it. Although vaccination has not been very hi-tech by present standards, small pox is the only disease that we have been able to eradicate to this day. He credits vaccination to be the highest technology in medicine.

Edward Jenner gets all the credit for discovering vaccination. Interestingly enough, an audit today would show him in very bad light; not by any stretch of imagination would what he did then have passed the ethical committee norms of today.

One of the Fellows of the Royal College of Physicians of London, JZ Holwell, FRS studied the wisdom of India in the eighteenth century by going there and remaining there for some years along with twenty other Fellows of the Royal Society. The Royal Society had sent some of its Fellows to study the science and technological developments in that subcontinent in the distant past. All those reports of the Fellows have been brought out recently in a book form by the Academy of Gandhian Studies in Hyderabad. Prof Dharmapal in this book *Indian Science and Technology in the Eighteenth Century* has given a graphic description of the vaccination methods then prevalent, as noted by JZ Holwell, quoting from Holwell's original lecture in 1767 to the President and Fellows of the Royal College of Physicians of London:

"The art of medicine has, in several instances, been greatly indebted to accident; and that some of its most valuable improvements have been received from the hands of ignorance and barbarism; a truth, remarkably exemplified in the practice of inoculation of the small pox," was the opinion of the College at that time. But Holwell studied the system for nearly twenty years, using the "most scientific" prospective cohort study design, to come up with the following opinion that he placed before the august body of the College for their consideration:

"However justified you gentlemens' remarks may be, you will be surprised to find, that nearly the same salutary method, now so happily pursued in England (**howsoever it has been seemingly blundered upon**), has the sanction of remotest antiquity (in India), illustrating the propriety of present practice"

Every year before the epidemic of small pox starts in early summer, a group of vaccinators, a tribe of Brahmins who are delegated every year from different colleges of Bindoobund, Eleabas, Benares, etc., arrive all over the provinces, dividing themselves into smaller batches, reaching their destinations well before the onset of the epidemic. The local people, anticipating the arrival of this team, observe a strict regimen enjoined if they want to be inoculated. The Brahmins pass from house to house and ask if the inmates have observed the regimen enjoined and then start their work only on those that want to be inoculated. There is no compulsion; in fact, even the number of points they want to be inoculated at depends on the recipient's choice.

The outside of the arm is preferred. First, the operator takes a piece of fresh cloth, which becomes his perquisite if the patient is affluent, and cleans the arm area to be inoculated. It is dry massage for a good ten minutes. Then with a special lancet, which is much better than the one used in England, scratches the arm area thus cleaned without drawing blood. The chief of the team keeps a double rag linen bag in his waistband in which the previous year's pus from an inoculated pustule (**never from a patient suffering from the disease**) is preserved. This is then smeared on to the scratch and bandaged with clean cloth to be kept for a couple of days. Before closing the wound a few drops of Ganges water are poured over it. Throughout this procedure a mantra of worship for the female deity in charge of this disease is continuously chanted.

The pus used is from an inoculated pustule of the previous year, for they never inoculate fresh material, nor with matter from disease caught in the natural way, however distinct and mild the type might be. This is the best way of attenuating a live virus. Following the inoculation the person had to observe a strict regimen of diet and treatment for the mild eruptive fever that follows. Holwell wrote: **"Although I was prejudiced in the beginning and many practitioners modified the technique, based on their teaching back home, my follow up studies showed that the altered methods lost many patients and the Brahmins' methods did not lose any patient.** A follow-up showed that almost 90% of those inoculated escaped while 90% of the uninoculated died during the following epidemic!" Holwell has given detailed reasons why certain food items like milk and fish were prohibited and showed that it was based on very sound scientific reasoning.

The inoculated person got a very mild eruptive fever, which invariably settled down with another treatment regimen to be followed very strictly and the inoculated person thus became immune to the natural and almost fatal disease! Holwell quoted two of his predecessors who commended this practice as very accurate with invariable success and venerable antiquity for its sanction. They were Helveltius and Kirkpatrick.

The Heart and its Diseases

The following stanza in the Shushrutha Samhita, the most important text book in Ayurveda, clearly describes the pain of myocardial ischaemia (anginal pain) in such great detail that it cannot be bettered even now. The interesting aspect of the treatise is the reference to the cause of pain in the beginning of the stanza, viz., "hradrogam" (heart disease).

Although once called the English disease, angina has its first well-documented authentic description in Ayurveda.

Thrichatwarimshathammodhyayah

> *Athaatho Hradrogaprathishedam Vyakyaswamyah*
> *Yathovaacha Bhaghavan Dhanvantharim (suthruthaya).*
>
> *Aayammyathe Maaruthaje Hradayam Thudyathe,*
> *Nirmathyathe Dheeryathe Cha Spotyathe Paaticha*
> *Thrishnoshadaahachoshaam Syuhu Paithikecha,*
> *Dhoomaayanam Cha Moorchaa Cha Swedhahako.*

(In this chapter, Bhagavan Dhanvanthari, the God of healing, personally describes the symptoms of heart disease and impending death due to heart attacks. The patient may feel pricking pain, vibrations (palpitations), and burning pain, at times the pain may be very severe resembling the pain of splitting the chest into two halves with an axe! He may have unusual thirst, burning all over, breathlessness, extreme exhaustion, and mouth breathing because he cannot have enough breath through his nostrils, profuse sweating, pale face, stiffness of the body parts, and, finally, even unconsciousness may result!)

Heberden, an English physician, credited with the first authentic documentation of angina pectoris in the 18th century, gave a graphic description of his own chest pain, but had no idea that the pain came from the heart. His student, Edward Jenner, of vaccination fame, thought that his boss's chest pain was due to syphilis. It was only around 1905 AD that William Osler, a great medical brain of the last century, postulated that the chest pain that Heberden had could have been due to heart disease.

A reference has already been made to the accurate anatomical knowledge in Ayurveda. In the **Dashasookthaani**, there comes the **Narayansookthaani** mantra. These are derived from the **Yajurveda** originally. Three manthras, numbers 7–10, deal mainly with the anatomy of the heart and there is also a graphic description of the physiology in the **Naadigranthas.**

"Heart is said to reside in the chest between the neck and the navel, twelve finger-breadths above the navel. Although centrally situated it points slightly to the left of the midline. It is said to resemble a large lotus bud kept upside down with its tip to the left. A large vessel, in addition to many vessels in that region, arises from the heart and takes blood (God's power) to all parts of the body from head to the tip of the toe, keeping the whole body warm. The diameter of this large vessel is smaller than the inner diameter of the cavity of the heart!"

In the physiology section we are told that the heart contracts and relaxes on its own, actively pushing and receiving blood at the same time repeatedly without any break. **Even the receiving of blood is an active process according to this document**. Frank Starling did think that it was only possible for God to understand the complete working of the heart. He, therefore, could only partly comprehend the systolic function of the heart in formulating what we now call Starling's laws.

It is only recently that a New York based venous surgeon of Indian origin, Dr Dinker Rai, stumbled on the possible diastolic suction of the atria, while working on a dog which died in the middle of his experiment. Analysis of his venograms in retrospect, in the cine films, showed the dye jumping into the heart from the inferior vena cava, coinciding with the atrial diastole. He will soon be writing this up (personal communication).

Thousands of years ago, Ayurveda knew this truth!

Mind and Disease

That human mind plays a role in disease is a recent thought in modern medicine. The earliest document in this field is that of William Harvey (AD 1648) which goes thus:

"I was acquainted with another strong man, who having received an injury and affront from one more powerful than himself, and upon whom he could not have his revenge, was so overcome with hatred and spite and passion, which he yet communicated to no one, that at last he fell into a strange distemper, suffering from extreme oppression and pain of the heart and breast and in the course of a few years died. His friends thought him poisoned by some maleficent influence, or possessed with an evil spirit.... In the dead body I found the heart and aorta so much gorged and distended with blood, that the cavities of the ventricles equaled those of a bullock's heart in size. Such is the force of the blood pent up, and such are the effects of its impulse.... We also observe the signal influence of the affections of the mind when a timid person is arrested, a deadly pallor overspreads the surface, the limbs stiffen, the ears sing, the eyes are dazzled or blinded, and, as it were, convulsed. But here I come upon a field where I might roam freely and give myself up to speculation. And, indeed, such a flood of light and truth breaks in upon me here; occasion offers of explaining so many problems, of resolving so many doubts, of discovering the causes of so many problems, so many slighter and more serious diseases, and of suggesting remedies for their cure, that the subject seems almost to demand a separate treatise.... And what indeed is more deserving of attention than the fact that in almost every affection, appetite, hope, or fear, our body suffers, the countenance changes, and the blood appears to course hither and thither. In anger the eyes are fiery and pupils contracted; in modesty the cheeks are suffused with blushes; in fear, and under a sense of infamy and of shame, the face is pale, but the ears burn as if for the evil they heard or were to hear; in lust how quickly is the member distended with blood and erected!"

Many studies in the recent past have demonstrated the pivotal role played by negative emotions like anger, jealousy pride and depression in the causation of major degenerative diseases. A glance at the following stanza will convince one about the ancient eastern thinking in this field.

Khrodha Shoka Bhaya Aayaasa VirudhannaBhojana Thaponnalan, Katwaamla Lavana Theekshnonathi Raktha Pitta Prakopayeth

(Anger, sorrow, fear, exhaustion, wrong type of food, sedentary living, acidic diet, salt, too much of condiments in diet, will eventually lead on to all the disturbances in every system of the body.)

Since the Second World War the stockpiling of nuclear weapons has been going on at a breathtaking speed. That apart, there have been crises everywhere which could be gauged from the daily newspaper reports of unrest in every sphere of human activity, viz., unemployment, energy crisis, health care crisis, atmospheric pollution, change in the biosphere, alteration in global temperature with global warming, violence and crime on an unprecedented scale all over the world with special emphasis on terrorism, political unrest in many countries, some countries trying to come together while others break up, man killing man in the name of religion, caste, and creed, and man trying to destroy all the God given resources of this world for his greed.

I am afraid I must confess that this change in this century might be due to the so-called scientific temper of the mechanistic concepts introduced by Descartes and Newton of reductionism. In the name of science this world also is being split into bits and pieces. Max Bohm, the great guru of German physics, had warned us about the ominous significance of our pursuing the reductionist science as an end in itself. While his three Nobel Laureate students, Oppenheimer (American), Fermi (Italian), and Neils Bohr (Scandinavian), were trying to split the atom in the thirties he did warn us: "*I am very proud of my pupils' cleverness, how I wish they had used their wisdom in place of cleverness.*" He went on to add "*that little atom mankind is intent to split-will teach mankind a lesson one day.*"

Fritjof Capra, a noted American physicist, says it beautifully in his book *The Turning Point*: "The new concepts in physics have brought about a profound change in our world view; from the mechanistic conception of Descartes and Newton to a holistic and ecological view, a view which I have found to be similar to the views of mystics and sages of all ages and traditions.... The exploration of the atomic and subatomic world brought them (physicists) in contact with a strange and unexpected reality that seemed to defy any coherent description.... Scientists became painfully aware that their basic concepts, their language, and their whole way of thinking were inadequate to describe atomic phenomena.... It took them a long time, but in the end they were rewarded with deep insights into the nature of matter and its relation to the human mind.

The emphasis of the effect of the mind on the body is so great in Ayurveda that one finds a pivotal role for the mind in the causation of all diseases:

Prasanna aathma indriya manaha swastha ithyabhideeyathe.

(happiness of the soul, senses, and the mind would ensure good health for all times)

Human consciousness is the foundation on which rests the superstructure of the human body and its ramifications. Ayurveda correctly identifies mind as a quantum concept at the subatomic level, which pervades the whole organism. The latest concept of teleportation gives credence to this view. Ayurveda is a holistic science. Management of diseases in Ayurveda should, per force, take the patient's mental state into consideration first.

The science of Yoga in Indian wisdom does just that. "Chitta vritti nirodhaha yogaha"—if one could control the undulations in the mind he will lead a healthy life. The latest truth in modern medicine is seen here having been proclaimed thousands of years ago. There is a common saying that if you could keep a child's heart as you grow old you would live long. This has been shown elegantly in the breathing exercises of yoga (praanayaama) where the heart rate variability (HRV) with breathing is being controlled. The sinus arrhythmia of an infant comes back alive even in old age when one could practice this breathing technique. A very recent study published in The Lancet shows the great physiological advantages of this method even in severely ill patients with heart failure.

Future Predictions in Medicine

Having practised medicine for nearly four decades, I have come to believe that the reductionist science in medicine has come to naught. We have been barking up the wrong tree trying to predict the unpredictable future of the human organism. Professor Firth, a professor of physics in the Strathclyde University in Glasgow, in an article in the 1991 Christmas issue of the *British Medical Journal*, had elegantly shown how the linear mathematics used in medicine and the reductionist logic of splitting the body into organs has resulted in wrong conclusions. He rightly captioned his article *Predicting the Unpredictable.* He advocated the use of the new holistic view to the study of human body and its ills, using non-linear mathematics and the new science of CHAOS, which look at the whole.

It is the greed of the present day "scientific" man to be successful in competition that has put the world in this situation of confusion and turmoil. Man is born with only two instincts: that of self-preservation and procreation. All the other emotions like hatred, jealousy, anger, and pride are injected after birth by environmental influences, the most important being early schooling where the innocent child is taught all these ills of modern day society's "dog eat dog" philosophy. Socrates was right when he said, "Let not my schooling come in the way of my education". Today's education does just that. We seem to have forgotten the dictum of John Adams who said in 1644 "education is that process which makes man to act justly, skillfully, and magnanimously under all circumstances of war and peace".

In today's world justice gets subordinated to power—money power or muscle power, and sometimes, even to the scientific power of the atom bomb. Magnanimity is a thing of the past. The wisdom of yore in the East as also in West proclaimed to the world that the best way to live happily is to live with three qualities engrained within us: Justice, beauty, and equality, which are always there within us. If they could be brought to the surface this world would be a happier and healthier place to live.

Indian Ayurvedic Oath vis-à-vis the Hippocratic Oath

The Indian ethics of the medical profession are, if anything, much more elaborate than the Hippocratic Oath itself. The following is the oath of the Indian physician:

- You must be chaste and abstemious, speak the truth, and not eat meat.
- Care for the good of all living beings; devote yourself to the healing of the sick even if your life were lost by your work.
- Do the sick no harm; not even in thought seek another's wife or goods.
- Be simply clothed; drink no intoxicant; speak clearly, gently, truly and properly.
- Always seek to grow in knowledge.
- Do not treat women except their men be present; never take a gift from a woman without her husband's knowledge.
- When a physician enters any house he must pay attention to all the rules of behavior in dress, deportment and attitude.
- Once with the patient he must in word and deed attend to nothing other than what concerns the patient.
- What happens in the house should never be discussed outside; nor must he speak speak of possible death to his patient, if that might hurt him or anyone else.

In the face of Gods and man you can take upon yourself these vows; may all the Gods aid you if you abide thereby; otherwise may all the Gods and the sacra, before which we stand, be against you.

And the pupil should consent to this.

Research in Medicine

There is a world of difference in the research methodologies of the ancient Indian system and those of modern medicine, especially the epidemiological research. Research in Ayurveda has been of the prospective cohort study variety where the follow up observations have gone on for hundreds of years. Modern epidemiological studies mostly follow the short-term case control methods that have many built-in flaws. The latter, therefore, result in frequent changes in our ideas and advice to patients. Two examples would be sufficient to support this theory.

Years ago it was thought that the main fault in diabetes mellitus was the leakage of sugar, and patients were, therefore, advised to take large quantities of sugar. One could only imagine the damage that advice would have done. On realizing the mistake it was argued that instead of sugar they should take large amounts of fat to compensate for the lack of carbohydrates. This again must have resulted in many atherosclerotic deaths. Time was when a high protein diet was advised, only to be followed by the sane advice of a sensible normal diet, which needed to be tapered to the needs of the patient. Underweight diabetics eat more calories while the overweight ones cut down on their calories. The latter has been the advice in Ayurveda for thousands of years.

Our ideas about the diet for atherosclerotic diseases have ranged from no fat to low fat. All kinds of absurd ideas were popular in the field from time to time. While butter was a taboo a few years ago, the slogan later on was butter is better. Saturated fat to polyunsaturated fat was the advice till recently, but now reports are trickling in of the ravages of mainly polyunsaturated fats. Ayurveda had one advice, which seems the most sensible even today.

Ghritham thejasvinam, pittaanila haram, rasasoujasam.

(Ghee gives you good health, counteracts the bad effects of pitta and anila, and promotes well being.)

Indian melted butter (ghee) is supposed to be the best fat in diet, although in moderation. Scientifically, ghee is butter minus animal protein. It is just caprionic and butyric acids—the two most useful and safe fatty acids. Similarly coconut oil (fresh) was advised as the best cooking medium. Although it contains saturated fats it is composed mainly of medium and short chain fatty acids, again good anti-atherosclerotic fats. It says that cooking oils must be fresh. This is the best advice in that preserved oils and solidified oils get transformed into trans-fatty acids—the most dangerous ones for the blood vessels!

Life Style Changes and Health

The Indian system maintains that a change of life style is the best insurance against precocious diseases. The advice given is for all times:

**Nithya hita mita aahaara sevi, sameekshakaari,
Datha samaha sathyaapara, kshyamavaan,
Vishaye vasaaklthaha, aapthopasevi,
Bhaveth aarogyam.**

(Daily eat food in moderation but that which pleases you, work very hard, do not tell lies, cheat others, or backbite people, have the courage to forgive others, always post-judge issues, and treat everyone as your near and dear ones—you will always enjoy good health)

This would look very modern by the present standards, but has not changed in thousands of years. Modern medicine does not stress on these ideas very much and has been changing its advice on and off, although there had been a textbook of medicine written by Charles Scharschimdst way back in 1734 in Vienna, where he was the professor of medicine at a very young age of twenty-six, wherein he emphasized the need to change the mode of living to be healthy.

Modern Pharmacokinetics

While the reductionist science follows the dictum of splitting the organs into their cells and then studying their functions to study the drug effects on them, Ayurveda has been studying the effect of drugs on the whole system along with the environment.

Recent work seems to agree with Ayurvedic thoughts. A large study in Canada of the effects of antioxidant vitamins versus an extra intake of fruits and vegetables in a large cohort of postmenopausal women showed a marked benefit in the latter group. In an editorial, the *British Medical Journal* went on to say that there could be many other antioxidant factors in the whole fruits and vegetables, in addition to the known A, C and E vitamins in the tablets.

Similarly, an editorial in the *BMJ* entitled *Garlic is good for cooking but not for health* did take into consideration the fact that all the forty odd studies referred to therein, used garlic extract pearls or tablets and not fresh garlic as a whole. Garlic, to be effective, has to be chewed in the mouth raw where salivary enzymes convert the inactive principles into active ones before swallowing. In the pills and pearls the SH group, the heart of the antioxidant property of garlic as also its antiplatelet property, is removed to mask the smell! Garlic is supposed to be a very important medicinal tool in Ayurveda. Recent studies in Harvard reconfirmed the Ayurvedic truth that raw ginger along with garlic and pepper has the most potent antiviral antibiotics against Flu and other respiratory viruses!

One could go on and on but I hope I have made my point. Ayurveda is very authentic. It has had thousands of years of longitudinal observational prospective research to back its claims. We could further elucidate its different claims with the modern methods of inquiry, to separate the wheat from the chaff. It is very modern in that it has been using non-linear mathematics from the beginning. Modern medicine is just realizing the futility of linear mathematics in dynamic systems and is groping in the dark trying to use non-linear mathematics. David Eddy, a former professor of cardiac surgery at the Stanford University who now teaches mathematics at Duke University is trying to educate medical researchers in the correct methods of research.

FURTHER READING

- Lewis Thomas. *The Lives of a Cell* 1984. Bantam New Age Books, New York.
- Laxmikantham V. *Origin of the Human Past*. Bharathiya Vidya Bhavan, Bombay,1999.
- Kutumbiah P. *Ancient Indian Medicine*. Orient Longman's Bombay, 1962.
- Inge WR. *Religion in Legacy of Greece*. Clarendon Press. Oxford 1921. Page 28.
- Milan RM. Practice of Inoculation in the Benders Division. Report of the Superintendent General of Vaccination to Government of NWP; dated 6th June 1870. Pages:72–77
- Dashasookthaani. Narayanasookthaani (Kannada)
- William Harvey. Quoted by Inglis B ' *A History of Medicine'*, Cleveland. The World Publishing Company 1965; pp 179–180
- Whiteman MC, Fowkes FGR, Deary IJ. Hostility and the Heart. *BMJ* 1997;315: 379–380.
- Hegde BM. Mind and Disease. *'VHS Bulletin* Madras. 1986;XV: 14–18.
- Lancet Study. Breathing.
- Stuart E: Consciousness - a new meaning. *Proc Roy Coll Phy Edin*. 1997; 27:68–74.
- Firth WJ. Chaos - Predicting the unpredictable. *BMJ* 1991; 303:1565–1568.
- Hegde BM. *Hypertension-Assorted Topics*. Bhavan's Bombay 1993.
- Hegde BM: Chaos in Medicine. *J Assoc Phy India* 1996;44:167–168
- Fruits and Veg. BMJ Study. Garlic. BMJ study.
- Hopkins EW. *Religions of India*. Page 559, as quoted by Kutumbiah P (3)
- Kutumbiah P. Air, Water, and Places of Charaka Samhita. *Ind J Hist Med*:1960;5:9–18
- Smith R. Where is the Wisdom? *BMJ* 1991; 303:6806:798–799.
- Milan RM. Practice of Inoculation in the Benders Division. Report of the Superintendent General of Vaccination to Government of NWP; dated 6th June 1870. Pages:72–77

CHAPTER 49

What is Yoga and What is not Yoga?

Yoga Shastra, the science of Yoga, first enunciated by Sage Patanjali, is one of India's greatest contributions to the world, in the sphere of maintaining good health and peaceful living. This is once again the need of the hour today, in a world torn into pieces by hatred, greed, and strife. Yoga underwent many transformations over the centuries and is being practised in many different forms in other Asian countries. The west has received Yoga in a much distorted version, and Yoga has been made to appear very simple and easy in order to cater to the fast moving western life style, mainly to make money for the seller. Whereas Yoga is the panacea for the fast pace of life, its present *avatar* in the west might not serve the desired purpose.

Ayurveda, the great Indian medical wisdom, which is the mother of much other medical wisdom in the world, including modern medicine, was based on two basic principles viz:

Swasthashya swastha rakshitham.
(Try to keep the WELL healthy)

Prasanna Aatma, Indriya, Manaha Swastha Ithyabhideeyathe
*(Keep the mind and senses happy and tranquil:
good health will be guaranteed)*

Modern medicine has realized, to its utter dismay, that the above truths are scientifically correct even today. Recent studies, both in the US and

Europe, have brought to the forefront the confirmation that the most important risk factors for major killers are in the human mind. Hatred, jealousy, greed, and pride, coupled with anger, frustration, and depression are at the root of many, if not all, major killers. Yoga, in its true form, should then be the logical panacea for all major illnesses. Scientific studies in India, in the US and England have again reiterated the above fact that Yoga and lifestyle changes, based on the science of yoga, could even reverse many damages to the body, including blood vessel blockages!

The human mind, according to ancient Indian wisdom, has several levels of development. One could develop one's mind to the highest level, *Ishwara,* when one becomes almost divine in one's approach to life. In between, there is a level, *the Chitta,* where one brings his/her ego to work. All problems start when one brings greed into the picture.

Chitta vritti nirodhaha Yogaha
(When the mind becomes tranquil, one becomes a Yogi)

In essence, Yoga is meant to make the practitioner's mind tranquil under all circumstances of sorrow and joy. Although it looks like a tall order, for one who practices real Yoga on a regular basis, this state of mind is not difficult to achieve. How does Yoga achieve its objective? Let us have a scientific peep into its working in the light of modern science.

Yoga has eight limbs—*astaanga Yoga.* They are *yama, niyama, praanaayaama, prathyaahaara, dhyaana, dhaarana, samaadhi, and aasana.* A real practitioner will have to observe certain codes of conduct. Regular exercise, moderation in food habits, preferably a vegetarian sattvic diet, truthfulness in dealing with the world, overcoming desire for what does not belong to oneself, concentration and meditation, *praanaayaama,* the breathing techniques of various kinds, and Samadhi. The last simply connotes the state of mind that an authentic practitioner attains if he follows the other rules. *Aasanaas,* the various postures that are sold to the gullible public as the be-all and end-all of Yoga, are only meant to help one to attain constant ease, which is just the pre-requisite for practising the other seven limbs of Yoga. When one equates the postures, the *aasanaas,* to the whole science of Yoga, the result could even be counterproductive, although it is true that muscle stretching alone might produce mind calming endorphins from the muscles!

The most important part of Yoga is the breathing technique—*praanaayaama.* This, in short, is simple belly button breathing. Deep slow breaths make one fully use one's diaphragm, the muscular wall between the abdominal cavity and the chest. Normally, man uses only a small portion of the lung (say, 20%) in breathing. If one gets angry even that comes down to 10% and the rate of breathing becomes very fast with a faster heart rate as well to compensate for the lack of oxygen inside. All these make the oxygen exchange in the lung, between the atmospheric air breathed in and the unoxygenated blood coming from the right heart, less efficient. Deep slow breathing, the essence of *praanaayaama*, would immediately bring more than 90% of the lung area into action for oxygen exchange.

This quickly raises the tissue oxygen levels significantly. When every cell in the body, of which there are one hundred thousand billion in all, gets better oxygen supply, the body works very efficiently. This makes the human mind, situated at the sub-atomic level at every human cell, become tranquil automatically. This might sound esoteric to some but one only has to experience it to realize how easy it is for an ordinary person to attain that state of mental tranquility. Charlatans teach some other methods of breathing that might result in hyperventilation and give one a dizzy feeling. This dizzy feeling is sold to the gullible public as the real effect of Yoga.

Unfortunately, if one is past middle age and gets into this hyperventilating state, one could even die of a sudden heart attack—a true meeting with the Maker, in a manner of speaking. Hyperventilation brings on changes in the blood pH, resulting in alkalosis. The latter could produce severe constriction of blood vessels. If that happens in the heart or brain, the result could be disastrous, to say the least. Be warned; never try any other type of *praanaayaama*, other than the one described above; *sukha praanaayaama*, if you are not a mature Yogi of the highest order. This type of yogi can perform many other feats, like slowing his breathing and heart rates to abysmally low levels that would be fatal for ordinary mortals. We cannot realistically hope to attain those levels of the Yogis.

Conversely, if one becomes tranquil, the breathing automatically becomes deep and slow, just as in Yoga practice. The essence of Yoga, therefore, is true tranquility of the mind at all times and not just for an hour or so daily during Yoga practice. To that end, one must have a tranquil life-style which makes one a Yogi in the true sense of the word. Religiously practicing Yoga daily for an hour, then trying to be one-up on others for the rest of the time would be of no use at all. One must follow the true *Indian culture* to be good at Yoga practice. Yoga cannot be practised in isolation. **True Indian culture is genuine authenticity-not doing anything that one does not want the world to know.** This, coupled with altruism, concern for others in distress—*sarve janaaha sukhino bhavanthu* (may everyone be happy)—makes life a true joy. In short, if you live and let others live, life would be a bed of roses.

In the present day world of cut-throat competition, man has almost forgotten what happiness is all about. The time was when the joy of hard work to earn one's next meal was sheer delight. Today mass production of goods, coupled with aggressive marketing techniques, have taken that joy away for the rich and the powerful. It is still a joy for those that do not know where their next meal comes from. For the rich now, happiness is in one-up-man-ship. Power emanates from hoarding. And even though the rich are in the minority, in the present day world the less fortunate poor are being daily exploited by the rich and powerful, making their lives miserable. The centuries-old idea that the richer one gets, the more powerful he/she will be is only an illusion. It remains a mirage even to this day.

To get rich, people use unscrupulous means. Truth and ethics become the major casualties. Now the reader would realize the greatness of the Indian culture *of not doing anything that one does not want the world to know*. It is in the pursuit of imaginary happiness—of hoarding—that man's breathing changes to the fatal mode, creating all the maladies that man has become heir to these days. In addition to trying to sell the modern medical *quick fixes* for the already broken glass of human health only for what they are worth in an emergency, one needs to go in for long term solutions of preserving the glass intact. In the end, health preservation is cheaper in the present medical care system, which has become prohibitively expensive with the greed of those that want to market their products and their skill. Yoga leads the way.

FURTHER READING

- "Wavelet Analysis of Heart Rate Variability: New Method of Studying the Heart's Functions: *Kuwait Medical Journal:* Sept. 2002: 34(3) : 195–200 : Rajendra Acharya, B M Hegde, Subbabba Bhat P, Ashok Rao, & Niranjan U Cholayya.
- Hegde BM. "Where is the Reality?" *Kuwait Medical Journal* 2002:34 (4): 263–265
- Hegde BM. Reductio Ad Absurdum. *Bull Royal Coll Physicians and Surgeons of Glasgow* 1997; 26:10–12.

CHAPTER 50

Health Scare System

The present day medical world is an enigma. I think the right name for the present system, which proclaims to *care* for the common man, would be *medical scare system,* as its main thrust is to scare the hell out of the common man. One example is enough. Whereas any lump in the breast has a *one-in-ten* chance of being malignant in India, every literate Indian woman gets bombarded daily with scary advertisements in so-called "*health*" magazines and news papers that unless she gets herself screened regularly she has a very high risk of dying from breast cancer. Nine times out of ten, a lump in the breast is not likely to be cancer and does not *harm* the owner! If this information is correctly disseminated, a lady with a breast lump might not die of fear. Fear does kill! This applies to other parts of the globe as well. No one bothers to tell the common man that drinking clean water could save more lives in poorer countries compared to all the cancer deaths put together. Only long experience in dealing with human suffering resulting from this kind of scare mongering would make one realize the gravity of the problem. Others might think this is only a minor aberration in the system, if at all.

Cancers grow very slowly, taking as long as ten to twenty years before showing up clinically. It takes years for the seed of any cancer, the *rogue DNA*, to multiply and mature to show up as a lump, etc. Cancer is caused by a defective *suicide gene*, which normally assists an ageing body cell to die by *apoptosis* at its appointed time, instead of letting the cell outlive its life span and mutate to become a rogue DNA. In that long interval, this "baby" cancer would die most of the time, if only one could make the environment inside one's body hostile for the cancer to grow. Happiness of mind and a frugal diet, mainly of fruits and vegetables, coupled with exercise, makes life miserable for the growing cancer cell, while a fat loaded, high calorie diet, coupled with mental frustration and depression, does help the cancer cell to multiply and grow very fast.

Truth is bitter and does not influence people easily. In the present medi-business it is not a good idea to make the common man complacent about his future. We, in the medical world, spend most of our waking time in predicting the unpredictable future of man, based on the patchy information that we get of his dynamic wonderful body, without having any inkling into his genotype or his mind. The latter two make up around 70% of man. "Future predictions are possible in dynamic systems only when one could know the *total initial state* of that organism", writes Professor William Firth, a great physicist, in the *British Medical Journal* of December 26th, 1991. Yet, doctors predict the unpredictable immediate and distant futures of their patients daily. The reasons are not far to seek. There are a host of connected businesses that will thrive and make profit from this scenario. The diagnostic centre, the mammogram manufacturers, the middlemen selling the equipment, the ancillary industries that feed the main plant making the mammogram, the financial institutions that fund the whole business, and, of course, the doctors and hospitals. No one dares to destroy the "rice-bowl."

If one could be certain about one's future, this world would be a miserable place to live, indeed. Nature, in its wisdom, kept the future of man uncertain, so that he could live with hope and be happy. Imagine a world where the future and one's death are all certain. Dr Herbert Nehrlich, an Australian physician, writing in the *British Medical Journal* of the August 18, 2004, opines thus about this:

"If we are going to be able to learn when we will have to put (as the Germans say) "the spoon down" then we will, hopefully, be advanced sufficiently to order replacements to carry on the tradition as well as the family name. I am talking about clones.

Imagine if we were to know the exact date of our death. How would we live our lives? Would the world be a better place, would we be nicer to each other? Would there be any need for doctors?

The Pharma Industry would surely hate it as no one would see the need for drugs, for screening or for the other shenanigans of what Professor Hegde calls the "Health Scare System". No more joggers, gymnasiums, but plenty of cigarettes, booze and recreational drugs. Unprotected sex, parachuting without a chute and swimming among the sharks would become routine. But no more wars! (Get shot today and live to tell the tale.) As to everyone carrying their own computer and determining genetic desirability or feasibility before any mating can take place, this is certainly nothing new at all. Adolph Hitler was into this head over heels. He would (and did) (in his own words) "wipe the slate clean". "Mental misfits", "sexual perverts" (e.g., homosexuals) and other genetically undesirables would be (and were) exterminated. He called them "sub-humans" (Untermenschen). Screening is a double edged sword. Antenatal screening presupposes that responsible people are the norm."

"To believe that doctors and hospitals help keep people healthy is plain rubbish," wrote MacFurlane Burnett. *How to avoid modern medicine*? was the title of an article written by Lord Platt in the early 60s. "More people make a **living OFF** hypertension than **die OF** it," wrote Sir George Pickering, a former Regius Professor of Medicine in Oxford, who also taught for sometime at Johns Hopkins. Sir George further wrote that anti-hypertensive drugs robbed the patient of all that is enshrined in the American Constitution (Thomas Jefferson 1772) of "life, liberty and pursuit of happiness." "Life", Sir George said, "we are not sure of, liberty the patient does not have, and happiness would be a thing of the past after he starts anti-hypertensive drugs!" This prophetic statement has now been ratified by newer studies that showed that many of the complications in those hapless patients are brought on by long term drug therapy and not by their elevated pressures! Old man Sir George must be having his last laugh in heaven!

Richard Asher, a great clinician who spent four decades teaching medicine at the Central Middlesex Hospital, London, wrote, "Riva Roci would grieve indeed, if he were to look at the abuse and misuse of the little box that he invented, which makes life miserable for human beings now" in his wonderful book *Talking Sense*. All this was long before the "HOT Study" and the ALLAHAT study. We are not told why the HOT (Hypertension Optimum Treatment) study was prematurely stopped and the results analyzed by the "intention-to-treat" method, while quite a few patients that started the study had dropped off by then because of intolerable side effects. Re-analysis of the famous UKPDS study showed how the authors were "seeing what they wanted to see" in the study. "Eye of the Beholder" is a good re-analysis of the "good" that bypass surgeries were supposed to do.

The CAST (Coronary Arrhythmia Suppression Trial) study showed that all that glitters is not gold in any drug arena. Statins are made out to be a panacea for all ills, while everyday a new dangerous side effect comes to light in the statin field, so much so that there is a whole web site devoted to the dangers of statins alone (www.thincs.org). Whereas there seems to be a pill for every ill, in reality, it is the other way round. **Every pill has an** ill, if not more, following it! **Pills could thrill but many of them surely kill in the long run.** A recent analysis of the immediate post heart attack revascularization showed that "getting admitted after a heart attack to a hospital with coronary bypass facility was the greatest risk factor (four fold increase) for strokes in the near future. This risk was much greater than hypertension, diabetes, etc.! Swan-Ganz catheters, albumin infusions, and, some key-hole surgeries have all come to grief sooner than expected. AIDS research is four times "richer" than cancer research and so is the retroviral drugs market! More and more people jump on the AIDS bandwagon these days than the numbers that get interested in cancer. No medical student gets to read the book *Inventing the AIDS Virus* by Peter Duesberg wherein a Nobel Laureate, Karry Mullis, the father of the PCR test that identifies viruses in the laboratory, questions the very connection between HIV viruses and the syndrome AIDS!

Good health needs very few things: clean drinking water, three square healthy meals, better sanitary facilities for the poor, clean surroundings, tranquility of mind, and moderate exercise on a regular basis. None of these are the concern of modern medicine. Health is our birth right. Our inbuilt immune system will keep us going as long as it can. In the unlikely event of it failing only should doctors intervene to "cure rarely, comfort mostly, but console always." Modern medicine's biggest curse has been "not letting the well alone." Screening the healthy for early diseases and intervening has been the bane of modern medicine, although it has been a boon to the industry. The safe bet for the common man would be not to go to a hospital when healthy. One should certainly see his/her doctor at the first sign of anything going astray with one's body or mind. The greatest discovery in science of this century is the discovery of man's ignorance. Our philosophers were not far off the mark. Michel Montaigne, the great French philosopher, put the idea in a nutshell thus: "Men are but vain authorities who can resolve nothing."

"Total body scan (TBS) is the most fashionable of gifts and perhaps particularly suitable for a 50th, 60th, or even 40th birthday. You might be giving your loved one the supreme gift of extra years of life. Unfortunately, you may be more likely to give him or her a lorry load of anxiety and a series of invasive, painful, and unnecessary investigations," says an advertisement.

Whole body scanning is currently being intensely marketed in the United States and the enthusiasm will surely spread. The "sell" is simple. You might have something horrible lurking in your body. The scan will show it and allow early treatment. Or the scan will give you the all clear, providing the perfect excuse for having paid an expensive dinner.

The problems lie in medicine's difficulties in defining normality, the devil of "false positives," and our limited understanding of the natural history of disease. The most common way of defining normal is that the measure lies within two standard deviations of the mean. So in a set of measurements from a normal population, 5% will be classed as "abnormal." The whole body scan will produce hundreds of measurements. So you have almost no chance of emerging as normal, but which of your abnormalities signify serious disease?

Stephen Swensen describes his experiences of using computed tomography to screen for lung cancer within the context of a major trial. His team has found 700 ancillary findings within its cohort, but most were false positives and led to "adversely affected quality of life" and "unnecessary diagnostic and interventional procedures."

AE Raffle and others analyze the outcomes of a form of screening that we understand much better, screening to prevent cervical cancer. They show that 1000 women have to be screened for 35 years to prevent one death. This means that one nurse performing 200 tests a year would prevent one death in 38 years. "During this time she or he would care for over 152 women with abnormal results, over 79 women would be referred for investigation, [and] over 53 would have abnormal biopsy results." During this time one woman would die of cervical cancer despite being screened. These authors also point out that over 80% of cases of high grade dyskaryosis and of high grade dysplasia do not progress to invasive cancer. The same may well apply in other organs, and the prophylactic removal of colons, ovaries, breasts, and gullets may be killing people without benefit." wrote Richard Smith, the then editor of the British medical Journal in his editorial (BMJ; 326:26th April).

Now the reader can better appreciate what I wrote in the beginning of this article concerning the natural history of cancers. If a cancer takes decades to manifest finally, where is the urgent need to scare the whole population about cancer screening? Early screening, done in order to improve cancer treatment, should aim at screening a person when the single cell outlives its time! This is humanly impossible, as all of us have a cancer or two starting in us everyday. Most, if not all, of them die a natural death, depending on our life style and mental equanimity. If one were to worry about the possibility of cancer death, he or she should get himself/herself screened everyday even if the medical world discovers a method of detecting the mutated rogue DNA in the body as it is born!

Medical science is based truly on the "Doctrine of Probabilities" of Blasé Pascal and not on the faulty "Laws of deterministic Predictability" of Isaac Newton. We would, however, like our patients to believe that medicine is a deterministic science. **Medicine, in reality, is only a statistical science. No scientist worth his salt would accept statistical science as pure science.** Everything is based on statistical methods and models. Statistics do not help the single, individual patient. Statistics apply to groups of individuals. A patient sitting across the table from the doctor with his/her problem could only be helped by the doctor's wisdom, vision, and past experience—not by statistical calculations. One would shudder to know that a recent *Institute of Medicine* report in the US, quoted by Barbara Starfield, in her commentary in the leading medical *Journal of the American Medical Association* (2000; 284: 483-485), showed that the third most important cause of death in the US is the medical establishment—doctors and hospitals—after heart attack and cancer in that order of importance.

Does the reader now want to believe that everything we do is based on altruism? It is very important to stress here that modern medicine is a panacea in any emergency, surgical or medical. The medical world has succeeded in relieving pain, the biggest enemy of mankind, under all circumstances. Mankind should be grateful for that. We doctors have a great responsibility when intervening in anyone that comes to us with any kind of suffering, even if knowledge in that field is equivocal. We have advanced to the stage of even transplanting damaged organs. Advances in disease management have been phenomenal in the last half a century. If only doctors leave the "well" alone, we will be shown as people who try to save human lives. The *Institute of Medicine* report, reported earlier in the chapter, would be reversed in our favour.

Medical community will not be able to change the future of man on this planet. We have not increased human life span, but have increased life expectancy, mainly because of better food, cleaner surroundings, education, and economic empowerment of the masses. The future medical world should avoid interfering in the lives of those that are well and productive. We should stop playing God to keep people alive here forever. We will never succeed. There are certain inflexible laws of Nature that man can't change. Science is only trying to unravel nature's mystery. Nobody invents anything in science; we only discover the secrets of nature. That should make all of us humble.

FURTHER READING

- Peter Duesberg. *Inventing the AIDS Virus*. 1997. Regnery Publications.
- Richard Smith. The Screening Industry. *BMJ;* 2003; 326 (26th April): 889
- Barbara Starfield. Is US medicine the best in the world? *JAMA* 2000; 284: 483–485.

CHAPTER 51

Medical Education in India

Medical education in India is based on the British model brought to India by the East India Company in 1857. Much water has flowed under the Howrah Bridge since, but not much has changed in the content and methodology of medical education in these one hundred odd years. We claim to have made significant changes in the last two decades, but most of it has been in cutting a little here or adding a little there, but comprehensive changes are the need of the hour. We still teach students within the four walls of the class rooms and the hospital wards, giving them very little exposure to the real world of illness and wellness in the community. The filtered serious and chronic or end stage diseases are being shown as the total spectrum of illness. Real world medicine has to be taught in the community set up.

Doctors are really trained to keep the health of the society and not only to make money by using technology and drugs. Unfortunately, students are taught very little about preserving the health of the "well" in society. The present "disease-based" medical education has to change to "patient-based" education, which I have labeled as medical humanism. It is the need of the hour. Humanism is a neologism that stresses the primacy of man in every thing that one does in society. Medicine revolves round anxiety—patient anxiety of disability and death and the doctor anxiety of "do I do more?" or "have I done the right thing?" If one could find a remedy for these two anxieties mankind would be happier. The route to achieving that goal in medicine is to train doctors to be human and humane to begin with and to train them to practise their craft with the utmost compassion for the hapless suffering people. Suffering could be due either to real illness or imaginary illnesses. Both need delicate handling. Doling out a verdict—"your heart is normal"—after a battery of expensive tests, does not allay the anxiety of a man who has come to find out 'what is wrong with him' in the first place. Medical ethics is no different from human ethics. Do unto others as you would like to be done to you.

In the last fifty odd years, technology has overtaken bedside medicine. Students normally do not learn much from what the teacher preaches but they learn more from what the teacher does. Seeing the "star performers" and the "thought leaders" use hi-tech gadgets both for diagnosis and management, the young students' mind absorbs the idea that good medicine can never be practised without those gadgets. **This is the reason why many, if not all our medical graduates, will not be able to practise in a village.** A conscientious student would feel guilty for not having had the benefit of the hi-tech stuff for diagnosis in the village and wants to shun village life altogether. This has resulted in the "inverse-care law" of medical practice. Whereas there is a dire need for good doctors in the villages there are very few and where there is already a surfeit of doctors in the larger metropolis still more are being added daily to compete in the new medi-business.

Be that as it may, the new graduates will have no idea about the common minor illness syndromes that form the bulk of societal illness burden! A study in Europe showed that the biggest cause of sick absenteeism is the feverish cold caused by an adenovirus. I am sure a new doctor would not have heard that name. Over the years with specialties growing and mushrooming, the poor graduate student is at the receiving end of the burden. Today a student has to pass an examination in every specialty, if not in the subspecialties. Information overload has made the textbooks too heavy. Memorizing those factual data to pass the end-year examinations, which we still follow in India, takes away both the joy of learning as also the essence of medicine, the doctor-patient relationship. One has to master the art of doctor-patient relationship in the earlier years at medical school. While the students have their bedside posting they would have one or the other of the Para-clinical end-year examinations looming large and distracting his/her total dedication from bedside learning.

All this could change if we make efforts to incorporate problem-based learning as also stressing on the methodology rather than the minutiae of information in the field. Most of the latter will have changed by the time the student graduates. That keeps changing after that too at a phenomenal speed. The problem with most of us would be not knowing which part of what we had learnt has, in fact, changed! Higher education should concentrate on methodology and leave the substance, which keeps changing, to the student to learn for himself/herself. Methodological expertise would enable the student to learn throughout his active life, the real continuing professional development. It has become very easy these days with advances in information technology.

Another problem is the mushrooming of medical schools in India in the last two decades. Most of them are "self-financing", a new label coined to cover the business that goes on in the name of education. All of them are not bad. Some are very good, indeed! Having said that, I must add that efforts in the non-governmental set up, especially in the higher education, are a dire need in India. With the demographic predications for the next fifty years we would need many more institutions compared to what we have today. Even now, India lags way behind many other countries. To give an idea, England has 353 Universities for a population of about sixty million, whereas India, with the population of 1.2 billion, has only 295 Universities. To have parity with England we should have around 6500 Universities today. No government will be able to meet the needs of more than 700 million young men and women knocking at the doors of institutions of higher learning in the next fifty years from the tax payers' money. Private initiatives are a need of the hour. It is estimated that our population in the next fifty years would have 70% below 20 years of age.

The need for more medical schools is real. The problem would be to keep up the standards. The present system of having an apex "watch-dog" body under the governmental control would be inadequate for reasons more than one. Power, that too absolute power, corrupts absolutely and makes life difficult for the honest players in the field. **This has nothing to do with individuals that hold high offices, but the very system has enough room for corruption, even if the people at the top are honest**. We need an independent body of medical educationists that have spent all their lives in this field to do this job without the government breathing down their necks. I could draw a parallel from the Flexner Committee that went into the status of the mushrooming medical schools in the US in the early 50s. They did a wonderful job to quietly separate the wheat from the chaff. The latter died a natural death in the years that followed leaving only the good ones to flourish even to this day. Similar effort must be made to keep a constant vigil on the quality of medical education in India. Being the buyer's market today students and parents would leave the bad ones alone to die a natural death without the government having to do the unpleasant surgery: which many times could be political suicide for the powers-that-be.

The parents of prospective doctors in the US, among the Indian Diaspora, would want this information to make up their minds before sending their wards to study in India. At the present time there are some agencies doing this job of ranking Indian medical schools; some of them publish their data in the leading journals in India. I must say that the grading is not done with rigorous scientific methodology, though. Teachers should make the student want to learn. There are many other good medical schools in India where one could send the children, but one will have to take the trouble to find out the conditions in the medical school they select. One would want to see, however, that all the schools come up to the expectations of the students and their parents.

The other lacuna in India is the need for medical schools to do more research. Clinical research need not always be expensive. Trying to find an answer to a bedside problem by going as far away from the bed as one could is, in essence, clinical research. This is lacking in India. I am not much concerned about the so-called "cutting-edge research" that people talk about. The latter involves sophisticated laboratories, expensive technology, large research grants, and competitive publications in the "prestigious" journals. Most of that is **repetitive** research. What takes knowledge forward in any field is not repeating known facts but **refuting false dogmas**. We in India, with our hoary past of great scientific wisdom, need to take advantage of that and do more and more **refutative** research and not waste our scarce resources in repeating what the western reductionist science is doing.

But it is not easy to get this message down at the present atmosphere of the lure for research grants etc. Very few organizations would come forward to fund refutative research. I have not been able to fully succeed in this venture in our own University although I am sure the seeds that I have sown will sprout one day and grow big. This kind of reductionist research has very little significance in the dynamic human body which does not follow the reductionist rules of linear mathematics.

Ayurveda has the best scientific method of classifying human beings into different genetico-constitutional types. This could help improve the randomized controlled studies (RCTs) of modern medicine. People belonging to the same type could then be matched for better results of controlled studies. The present RCTs are flawed. Time evolution in a dynamic system depends on the total initial state of the organism. The present matched controls are anything but identical and so the initial conditions are not matched. Long term outcomes of all the controlled study results are flawed now. Ayurveda could help medical research in a big way. Let us not go into the intricacies here as the scope of this chapter is different.

Modern medicine has become prohibitively expensive with modern technology. While modern hi-tech medicine is a must for emergency care it might be kept away from chronic incurable and minor illness syndromes to cut the total cost drastically and make medical care available to the poor also. This could be done by proper research to integrate the great Indian wisdom of Ayurveda, another allopathic system, as a complementary system along with modern medicine in Indian medical schools. This takes courage on the part of the powers-that-be as also effort by the medical leaders in the field of education to research the need to weed out the untested claims of charlatans practising the art of Ayurveda.

The great science of Ayurveda needs to be tested using the modern scientific methods to bring out the best to be incorporated in the new integrated medical curriculum. Much needs to be done in the area. Indian medial education has a very bright future and it could lead the rest of the world in its innovations if it gets out of the present delusion of following the ancient British model. Sooner it is done the better for mankind.

Men are vain authorities who could resolve nothing.

—Michel De Montaigne

FURTHER READING

- Hegde BM: Our Medical Education. *Indian J Medical Education.* 1991; XX (3): 1–4.
- Hegde BM: Probity in Medical Science. *J Ind Med Assoc* 1992:90:166–167.
- Hegde BM: Graduate Medical Education - Reappraisal. *JIMA.* 1992:90:205–207.

CHAPTER 52

How Might the Benefits of Ayurveda be Combined with Modern Medicine?

Philosophy

Ayurveda, the science of life (Ayu=life; vid=science) is a part of the ageless Vedic heritage of India. Speculations about its origin go back thousands of years before Christ. Extensive literature on this subject, dating back to the fourth century BC, has one thing in common that the essence of Ayurveda is to preserve good health, which is every human being's birthright. Ayurveda prescribes life style changes with emphasis on tranquility of mind that is filled with universal compassion, as an insurance against an occasional illness. In this system, disease is only an accident. Just as road accidents are rare if one follows traffic rules, disease would an exception if one follows the life style prescribed in Ayurveda, which is not hard to comply with.

Human body has an inbuilt powerful immune system that could correct most, if not all, ills that man is heir to. In the unlikely event of this mechanism failing, and only then, should doctors interfere to help the system, when possible. In fact, the concept of immune deficiency syndromes had been prevalent there. Immune boosting methods are the mainstay of Ayurvedic therapeutics, the *panchakarmas,* and the five modalities.

Swasthasya swastha rakshitham
(Keep the well healthy as long as possible is the motto)

This motto would be a great help to modern medicine where a stage has come, what with the array of scopes and scanners, coupled with our inability to define normality precisely, we end up with having no normal healthy human beings at all. Among the many methods of preserving health in Ayurveda, the one that stands out is Sage Patanjali's *Yoga Shashtra*, the science of Yoga. Unlike what is sold by the new age gurus, original Yoga had eight wings: rules for day-to-day living including diet, the art and ethics of living, regular exercise menu, the all important breathing method (*pranayaama*), detached outlook towards life, yogic postures for constant ease to enable one to practice the next steps of dhyaana—concentration, tranquility of mind, and the ultimate realization of the impermanence of life to make man fearless even in the face of death. Thus defined, Yoga becomes a way of life and not just a few contortions of the body for an hour or so daily. Yoga, in its true form, is a way of life.

Another distinct philosophy in Ayurveda is that every disease begins in our thoughts (consciousness) and grows in the body. Genetic contributions are very clearly understood, in addition. The concept is holistic and never reductionist. Man is a part of the Universal consciousness, the environment and even the stars are supposed to have a role to play. Modern medicine is just trying to grapple with the role played by the mind in serious illnesses. Science, especially quantum physics, seems to be going into the new realm of human consciousness. Werner Heisenberg's *Uncertainty principle* and Ervin Schrodinger's *Cat Hypothesis* point in that direction. Recent studies of patients revived after cardiac arrest and those undergoing brain surgeries have pointed to the possibility of human consciousness (mind) without the brain in every single human cell. This all-pervasive consciousness has been the hallmark of Ayurvedic thinking.

Effectiveness of Ayurveda

In the absence of its recognition by the mainline science journals, the studies in the field of Ayurveda find it very difficult to get published, but there have been modern scientific enquiries into the effects of Yogic breathing. Millions all over the world now practice breathing methods for good health. It has become another big business with all market force trappings. Small pox, the only scourge that we have been able to eradicate so far, was eradicated with the help of vaccination. The authentication for Edward Jenner's anecdotal experience came from the prospective controlled study observations of a London physician, TZ Holwell, FRCP, FRS, who after studying Indian vaccination systems prospectively for twenty long years in the Bengal province of the Raj, reported his findings to the President and Fellows of the London College in 1747. He wrote that the antiquity and the authenticity (ninety percent protection of the vaccinated) could certainly give credibility to Jenner's method. The graphic descriptions of the Indian method and its efficacy are portrayed in his paper, which could be viewed in the archives of the College library even today.

Although slightly damaged by the great London fire of the eighteenth century, the document, providentially, survived the fire to show the original method that eventually led to the eradication of the greatest scourge of mankind. Recent evidence also suggests that the mind could initiate the cardiac rhythm and also the arrhythmias.

Ayurveda classifies human beings into three distinct types, *vaata, pitta, and kapha* with multiple subtypes. This typing takes into account the phenotypical and geno typical features, in addition to consciousness. In short, it is a holistic concept, unlike the modern medical method of matching groups for controlled studies based on tiny fractions of the phenotype, like height, weight, age, sex and body mass index with a few of the biochemical and physical characteristics. This kind of science of reductionism has led to doctors predicting the unpredictable. An experienced Ayurvedic physician could classify his patients based on these types since the treatment modalities are individualistic and not based on controlled studies as in modern medicine. Each patient needs individual titration of the methods used for him. Since time-evolution, in a dynamic system, depends on the total initial state of the organism, controlled studies could be done using these personality types to match cohorts for better results in future. There are computerized systems to classify people based on this system.

Holistic Concept of Ayurveda

Ayurveda does not look at the human body as a sum total of the organs. The physiology in Ayurveda takes into account every aspect of man's existence, including the planetary influence. There is a whole science of Ayurvedic astrology. The various rhythms of the body like the circadian and ultradian were explained by their mode-locking to the most dominant rhythm of breathing. Breathing could control all the systems in the body except the one rhythm that occurs outside twenty-four hour cycle—the menstrual cycle that occurs once in twenty-eight days. This, Ayurveda, claimed is under the gravitational pull of the moon stimulating the human brain!

Kujendu hetu prathimaasaarthavam
(Because of the moon the woman menstruates once a month)

This might have looked very odd but for the fact that recent advances in human physiology have shown that the final stimulus for the endocrine orchestra that maintains the infradian rhythm of menstruation comes from the gravitational effect of the moon on the cortical cells.

Most of the present day "so-called" Ayurvedic drugs in the market are reductionist in that they are only the extracts of the active principle in the plant to conform to the modern medical standards of drug sales. *Dravyaguna*, Ayurvedic pharmacodynamics, does not deal with active principles. It deals with the whole plant extract as envisaged in the ancient texts. This takes into effect even the photodynamicity of the plant. Some plants are to be harvested only after sunset lest their properties should change if harvested while the sun is up. Modern medicine now tells us that extracts might have serious side effects in the long run. Vitamin C in large doses, over long periods, could encourage cancer growth in the body, but eating tomato daily with lots of vitamin C in it, would not harm the body. There are many unknown chemicals in the whole plant that prevent the active ingredient from harming the patient while, at the same time, potentiating the good effects of the active principle. We will have to standardize the drug delivery methods to conform to the present standards but on the basis of holism only. In fact, herbal medicines are the least important part of Ayurvedic therapeutics. While yoga, panchakarma, and surgery are the main stay, herbal medicines are occasionally used. Ayurvedic surgery was so advanced that the rhinoplasty method used by the Ayurvedic physician, Shushruta, is being used by plastic surgeons even today. His anatomy classes lasted more than two years for students and he had devised most of the important emergency surgical methods.

What should an Ayurvedic Doctor Do?

His main job is to study his patient in great detail with special reference to his surroundings and classify him. Having done that he should then try and tailor the management strategies. Most of them would need panchakarma methods. Almost all of them would do well with change of mode of living that ayurveda prescribes with special emphasis on diet, yoga, and exercise. Rarely do surgical methods and/or drugs become appropriate. With advances in modern science and technology one cannot ignore the benefits of using modern hi-tech methods for emergency care. This requires the conventional ayurvedic doctor to have a reasonably good knowledge of the modern medical methods to be able to give proper advice to patients. A judicious combination of modern medicine and ayurveda would be an ideal training for a family doctor. More skilled specialists in either system could be used only at the referral point. This would bring down the top-heavy cost of modern medical care remarkably.

More than eighty per cent of the illnesses are either minor or self-correcting. They could easily be helped using ayurvedic methods and a placebo doctor. In addition, Ayurveda could help chronic debilitating diseases to a great extent, at a very small cost to the taxpayer. About ten per cent of the time, modern medicine becomes mandatory. Roughly ninety per cent of the unnecessary cost could be reduced for the benefit of all without detriment to public health. Rather, most of the iatrogenic problems could thus be avoided. Iatrogenesis is usually due to the long-term side effects of modern drugs. The latter form about fifteen per cent of hospital admissions. Modern medical doctors, who do not have an idea of Ayurveda and how it works, could be baffled when confronted with a patient who has probably taken the wrong advice from unscrupulous ayurvedic practitioners. The whole gamut of these intricacies would have to be thrashed out before changing the system of medical education into a complementary holistic system.

Ayurveda would not be of much use in an emergency. For the management of emergencies we have to follow the modern medical methods. But for all the chronic degenerative and ageing problems, Ayurveda is a panacea. The cost is very small in comparison. Modern medical drugs and interventions are good for acute emergencies, but in the long run most of them have run into serious problems.

FURTHER READING

- Strandberg TE, Salomaa VV, Naukkarinen VA, et al. Long-term mortality after 5-year multi-factorial primary prevention of cardiovascular diseases in middle aged men. *JAMA* 1991 Sep 4; 266(9): 1225-9.
- Pimm vL, Ruud vW, Meyers V, & Elfeferich I. Near-death experience in survivors of cardiac arrest: a prospective study in Netherlands. *Lancet* 2001; 358: 2039-45.
- Greyson B. Dissociation in people who have near-death experiences: out of their bodies or out of their minds? *Lancet* 2000; 355: 460-63.
- Sabom MB. Light and death: one doctor's fascinating account of near-death experience. Michigan: Zonderyan Publishing House, 1998: 37-52.
- Bernardi et al. Effect of breathing rate on oxygen saturation and exercise performance in CHF. *Lancet*; 1997;351:9112.
- Hegde BM. Vaccination in India. *J Assoc Physicians India* 1998; 47: 472-473.
- Firth WJ. Chaos-predicting the unpredictable. *BMJ* 1991; 303; 1565-1569.
- *Cecil's Textbook of Medicine* 2001, page 1202.
- Andersson OK, Almgren T, Persson B, et al. Survival in treated hypertension: follow up study after two decades. *BMJ* 1998 Jul 18; 317(7152): 167-71.
- McCormack J and Greenhalgh T. Seeing what you want to see in randomised controlled trials: versions and perversions of UKPDS data. United Kingdom prospective diabetes study. *BMJ* 2000; 320:1720-3.

CHAPTER 53

Holistic Lifestyle Changes for Wellness

> **Silence is a powerful enemy of social justice.**
> —*Amartya Sen*, Nobel Laureate

Illness and wellness are two sides of the same coin. Man is born with all the necessary in-built repair mechanisms to correct most, if not all, deviations in health and go on as long as he/she lives. "Do not try to live here for ever, you will certainly not succeed" said Bernard Shaw. He couldn't be more accurate scientifically. All our efforts to remain healthy should not aim at the impossible state of immortality. This repair mechanism, referred to earlier, is the basis of our immune system. However, a holistic look at man's existence on this planet gives us an idea of the role played by man's genes and environment, both of which are supervised by man's consciousness. In short, most illnesses start in our minds only to grow in the body, aided and abetted by the fertilizers like tobacco, alcohol, wrong food habits, and pollution in our environment; of course, modulated by our genes which, in turn, depend on the environment and the mind for their penetrance, as shown in Fig. 1.

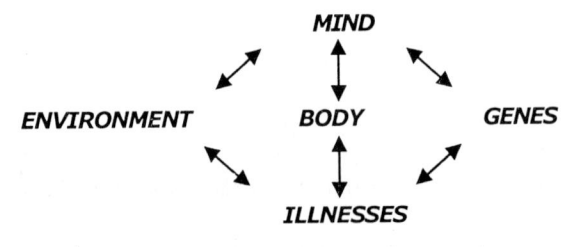

```
            MIND
              ↕
ENVIRONMENT ↔ BODY ↔ GENES
              ↕
          ILLNESSES
```

Fig. 1

Consequently, a holistic approach to healthy lifestyle will have to look into all these aspects of human life. Reductionistic ideas of lifestyle management where one or two of the above mentioned aspects are targeted will not bear fruit in the long run, although it might look fashionable in the beginning depending on how it is sold in these days of heavy advertisement. Correcting the body defects, like bypassing blocked vessels alone, does not change the overall outlook. **Minor changes in the initial state of an organism might not hold good as time evolves in a dynamic human organism. It might even be counterproductive as there could be the famous "butterfly effect" of physicist Edward Lorenz of weather predictions fame! Extremist views about drastic changes in diet also would meet the same fate for the same scientific reasons**. The *bija mantra* should be moderation in all aspects to have a salutary effect in the end.

Reductionism is the curse that medical science has inherited from the natural sciences of the 12th Century European Universities. Medicine has not kept pace with physics which changed direction in the early part of the last Century to follow the path of quantum mechanics. The latter with its understanding of the human consciousness, would be ideally suited to understand human physiology. The mind-body divide of the Cartesian *res cogitans* and *res extensa* has already done enough damage to the progress of medical science. **Holistic science of fractals, chaos, and non-linear mathematics would give respectability and credibility to medical research in the future**. This would necessitate us to look at human physiology, in health and disease, through the holistic glass.

Human Mind

Since all ills originate in the mind, time has come to think of keeping the mind healthy to have good bodily health. How to keep the mind clean? Modern medical research has already thrown enough light on the role of the mind in major killer diseases like heart attacks and cancer et cetera. Depression seems to be the major risk factor for cancer; depression and, most importantly, hostility have come out as the leading risk factors for myocardial infarction; anger is leading others in the race to get the credit for bringing on haemorrhagic stroke. Be that as it may, how do we alter this mental state? There have been attempts to alter the mental states of depression etc., using drugs with questionable change in the risk status.

Indian Ayurveda, the science of life, which has existed for "times out of mind" has understood the mind at various levels of development (evolution) and has the right advice to change the mental states for better. The great science of *Yoga* is said to be the right solution. Mind has five levels: *manus, budhi, chitta, purusha,* and *ishwara*. Man could evolve to higher levels of the mind by his/her effort. Up until the level of chitta man's ego does not alter the mental state of universal compassion. It is the ego at the level of the *chitta* that makes man unhappy and brings sorrow in its wake. It is at this level *Yoga (chitta vritti nirodhaha yogaha)* is said to be very effective. In short, true *Yoga* makes the mind to go back to the universal compassion stage of mind of a child, where even the immune system is now known to get a shot in its arm.

One cannot get to this stage by doing various body contortions (*aasanaas*) sold in the west by nearly forty three different schools of "so-called" *Yoga*. Unfortunately, none of them profess the true *Patanjali Yoga* that transforms the devil in man into his true divine self. One has to practice this always and not the half hour of circus. *Bhagavad-Gita*, the essence of Indian wisdom, proclaims that if one were to become a true *Yogi*, one automatically changes his breathing rhythm to that of *praanaayaama*, the be-all and end-all of a healthy lifestyle. We have been working for the last three decades to scientifically validate the good effects of *praanaayaama* on the cardiovascular system.

The Heart Rate Variability (HRV), an indicator of heart health, is the yardstick used in these studies. This concept is based on the scientific fact that in the dynamic Universe, as in any dynamic system like the human body, the most dominant rhythm subserves all other less dominant rhythms. This is called "mode-locking" in physics. Breathing being the most dominant human rhythm, heart and other organs are mode-locked to breathing. If one knows how to have healthy breathing pattern, his other organs become healthy too. The healthy sinus arrhythmia of a child that disappears with man ageing and becoming selfish is the sign of good health in a child. Our study has gone a long way in proving this. If one could fill the mind with universal altruistic love there will be no place for negative thoughts in the mind at all.

Our Diet

Most of the advice that we get about our diet from the existing "scientific" literature is unscientific, to say the least. The essence of healthy living is moderation in food intake. There must be a wide choice of foods in the diet. Vegetarian food is healthier since man basically is a vegetarian. Five to six small meals a day would be ideal. The meals must get smaller as the day goes and the supper must be the smallest. Of the six, three could be fruit meals only. Fat is an essential part of our daily intake but must be kept below 20% of the total daily intake. Other than mother's milk the next best fat in food should be coconut (or other palm) oil. Deep frying anything is not advisable. The western myth of cholesterol is only a business proposition AND HAS NOTHING TO DO WITH HUMAN NUTRITION, in the words of a famous chemist. If one has a disease called familial hypercholesteraemia, one might need appropriate treatment for that condition. Barring which, diet plays a very insignificant role in cholesterol metabolism. Cholesterol is a vital need of the body for building body cell wall. Very low cholesterol levels predispose to cancer in a big way! The first ever Diet-Heart Study in Framingham showed that the two are not directly connected, way back in 1959, but the study did not see the light of the day in print. Curious are the ways of science in the west. John Bokris, a great chemist, the father of cold fusion method, has called reductionist science as *a western religion* in his famous book *The New Paradigm.*

Regular Exercise

Regular exercise is one of the most important parts of the lifestyle modification. This is very important for today's white collar professionals and our sedentary housewives. For the hard working labour class, exercise could be a curse. Simple daily walks lasting up to one hour would be the best that could happen to our health. This as the power to keep us as healthy as possible and avoid many a fatal illness. Overexertion and heavy physical exercise like jogging are not healthy. The best part of daily exercise is the pleasure that it gives for a person who takes time to enjoy Nature en route. However, it should not be an obsession. Even if done for four to five days in a week it is as good as daily exercise. Swimming is another good exercise for those that have the means. Walking in waist deep water could also be very good.

Tobacco and Alcohol

These are the two deadly enemies of mankind, thanks to the monetary economy that promotes these two. Let us pay our tribute to Sir Richard Doll, who, for the first time, connected tobacco smoke with lung cancer and later with heart disease against strong opposition from his own colleagues and seniors at that time that it almost cost him his good job at the Hammersmith Hospital. He died this year in London at a ripe old age due to a short illness. If we, as a profession, could fight to get rid of tobacco habit from the population we will have paid a real tribute to him. His soul would then certainly rest in eternal peace. Much water has flowed under the London Bridge since then in this area of smoking and health both for the smoker and for his companions (passive smoking).

Alcohol is another story of using science (reductionist) as the cover to sell all kind of falsehoods and half truths to the gullible public and propagate the idea that a small amount of alcohol, especially red wine, is good for health and is a heart tonic. The truth however, is very far from that belief. Although we do not have unequivocal evidence to say that small amounts of alcohol are bad for health, we have not even an iota of evidence to say that a small amount of alcohol in any form is good for health! The evidence brandied around is only statistical evidence and most readers would know how to use statistics to sell what you want to sell. Medical science is not a true science; it is only a statistical science: the latter is called science without sense in a book by the same title by a great American epidemiologist, Steven Milloy. However, large studies today have shown that teetotalers are better off compared to the mild drinkers and heavy drinkers are the worst. Same is the advice given by Ayurveda. Caraka says that people drink all kinds of alcohol and some even enjoy doing that, but if one wants to keep away from diseases, he better keep away from alcohol of any kind.

Bad Genes

Many of us are worried about our bad genes from our parents if they had suffered from any serious disease. This is another myth created by the reductionist science of medicine and the vested interests. If the parents have had precocious disease below the age of thirty five or so, then there is a good possibility of the genes creating problems for the progeny. However, gene alone cannot bring on any disease in anyone. Absence of a gene is an insurance against that disease, but the presence of the gene only indicates the possibility of that disease coming on. Any gene needs a conducive environment to penetrate and show its power (gene penetrance). If one makes the environment hostile to the gene, the gene will not be able to bring on the disease easily. That is where the diet and the other factors come into play; in short, one has to have a holistic approach even to the gene's presence. Left alone, the gene is powerless. There are now evidences to show that even the genes could be influenced by the mind as shown by the inventor of then jumping genes hypothesis, Barbara McClintock, the Nobel laureate botanist: primacy of the mind again.

In conclusion, one could easily understand that the human body works as a whole and not in bits and pieces. Human mind is in the driving seat for wellness as well as illnesses. Man has two powerful attractors in phase space, a dynamic attractor called health, and a static attractor called death, as shown in Figure 2. Since health is a dynamic state where every parameter and organ of the body keeps actively changing all the time, health is a more durable state. Even if man gets thrown out of the healthy chaotic state (Point **A** in the figure), the natural tendency, most of the time, is to get thrown back into the state of health attractor for which all the necessary technology is built into the repair mechanism by Nature, the immune system. Occasionally, if man gets thrown out too far into the phase space (Point **B** in the figure) nearer the static attractor called death, he/she might die. It is in this state of illness that man could suffer a lot and needs medical help to "cure rarely, comfort mostly, but to console always." Problem comes only when doctors intervene unnecessarily with drugs and surgery at the time when man is only thrown out of the healthy chaos temporarily into point **A** with a natural tendency to be attracted back into the healthy attractor. Doctors do play a very important part even in these situations if they use their placebo skills to encourage and empathise to help the patient to get back into the healthy attractor, which is the rule. Too much intervention here might increase death and disability as is shown by the IOM report in the US. Wellness, therefore, should be the motto of the medial profession. Healthy lifestyle would certainly keep one healthy until death.

##
STATIC ATTRACTOR

Static Attractor######################################
##

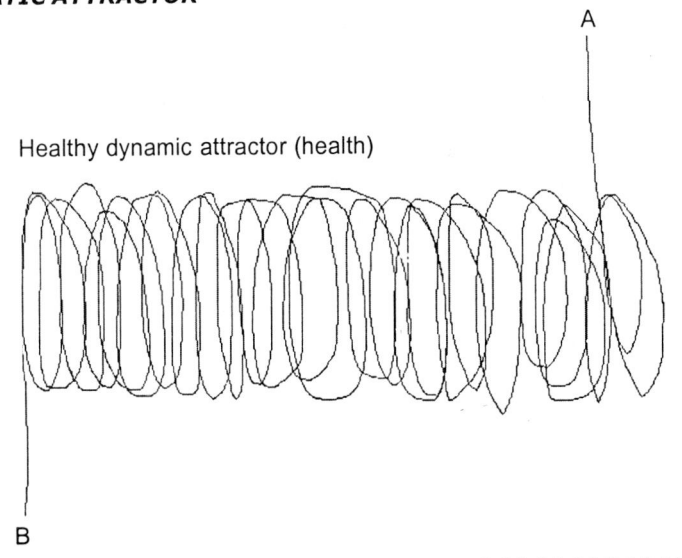

Fig. 2

"Tout passé, tout lasse, tout casse"
(Everything passes, everything wears out, and everything breaks.)
—*French Proverb*

FURTHER READING

- Acharya R, Hegde BM et al. Heart Rate Variability (HRV) - a non-linear measure *Kuwait Med* J 2003;35:208
- Bockris J. *The New Paradigm*. D&M Enterprises, College Road, Texas. 2005.
- Charles Townes. Of laser and prayer. *Science* 1997;277:891
- Firth WJ. Chaos-Predicting the unpredictable. *BMJ* 1991; 303: 1565-1568.
- Gribbin J. *In search of Schrodinger's cat*. 1991. Transworld Publishers, 61-63, Uxbridge Road, London W5 5 SA.
- Hegde BM. Need for a change in medical paradigm. *Proc Royal Coll Physi Edinb*. 1993; 23: 9-12.
- Hegde BM. The tyranny of prevailing opinion. *Indian Heart* Jr 1997;49: 439-441.
- Hegde BM; "Genes, Dreams and Realities" *J. Assoc. Physi. India* 1999; 47 (No.12): 1191-1193.
- Linden W, Stossel C, and Maurice J Psycho-social interventions for patients with CAD. *Arch Intern Med*. 1996; 156: 745-752.
- Milloy S. *Science without sense*. 1999. CATO institute, Washington DC.
- Ravnskov U. An elevated serum cholesterol is secondary, not causal, in coronary heart disease. *Medical Hypotheses* 1991;36:238-41.
- Sir Richard Doll. Obituary. *BMJ* 2005; 331: 295
- Romelsjo A and Leifmann A. Association of alcohol consumption and mortality, myocardial infarction and stroke in 25 years follow up of 49618 Swedish men. *BMJ* 1999; 319: 821-822.

CHAPTER 54

Hormesis – One Man's Meat is Another Man's Poison

The art of research is the art of the possible.
—*Peter Medawar*

Hormesis is the stimulation of any system by small doses of an agent which, in the larger doses, harms the same system. Hormesis (hormo in Greek= I excite) is a very important concept in science but, had been killed in its bud by the powerful people in science. Even a poison in small doses could benefit the human system. Hormesis is related to the word hormone, the chemical that stimulates many organ functions in the human body. Scientists think that Nature is foolish but, in fact, Nature is there to see that mankind and all other living creatures survive despite the environment being hostile, many times. The concept of hormesis is one of the reasons why homeopathic medicines work in many minor illness syndromes. In fact, modern medicine benefited from homeopathy in the discovery of nitrates in the treatment of anginal pain. In homeopathy, nitrates were used to treat headaches in small doses. Incidentally, nitrates reduced chest pain of angina in a patient who was taking the drug to relieve headache in the first place. Nitrates, in small doses, have the hormetic effect on headache while they bring on severe headaches in some patients when given in the "therapeutic doses" of modern medicine. One man's poison could be another man's meat.

Small doses of any drug possess a bio-positive effect while the large dose of the same compound has the opposite bio-negative effect. In short, all drugs have opposite effects in two dose extremes (see Figure 1). The young scientist that worked on this hypothesis for his PhD under the famous Stanford immunologist, George Fegan, to show that vitamin C could be dangerous in bigger doses while it is a stimulant and good for the health in very small doses never made it and had to leave science research altogether because Linus Pauling, the great hero of science, destroyed the young scientist completely. It was Pauling himself that had induced Fegan to work on the good effects of vitamin C on the immune system in the first place. The hormetic effect of vitamin C could not be swallowed by Pauling. Pauling could never agree with vitamin C being poisonous in larger doses! Later he fought an expensive legal battle against his own colleague, a former Director of the Pauling Institute, for showing that cancer growth is stimulated by vitamin C in larger doses, but Pauling lost the battle and was disgraced.

Pauling got the second Nobel (Peace) Prize, after his first for the discovery of vitamin C, by the same antipathy towards hormesis. Edward Teller was the father of American Nuclear deterrent against the communists. While Teller was testing atomic weapons, he showed the hormetic effect of radiation by accident. In very small doses radiation stimulates the immune system and increases human life span, radiation hormesis. It also slows the ageing processes by the hormetic effect of working as an anti-oxidant. This has been confirmed by the recent evidence that cancer incidence is less in areas around atomic plants as compared to normal populations.

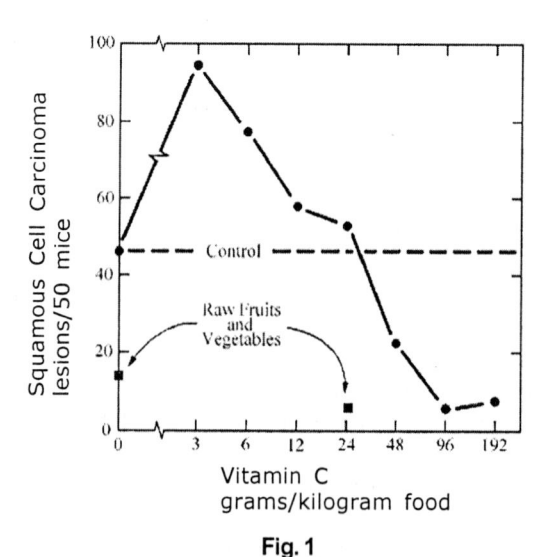

Fig. 1

The famous Teller-Pauling debates that followed took the whole of America by surprise. Pauling succeeded in demonizing Teller to the extent that the Swedish Nobel Academy gave Pauling the Nobel Peace Prize, his second Nobel! There are many such frauds that have occurred in science but, ordinary mortals do not come to know of them. Scientists have built such a great aura around them and the halo is so large that there are many who swear by the accuracy of science while the theta and delta faults make a mockery of most reductionist scientific discoveries. However, the technology industry has become a big money spinner and that feeds society with the myths about science. The recent study that daily intake of vitamins harms in the long run while fruits and vegetables help the human system greatly could be understood by the hormetic effect of vitamin C shown in the Figure 1. Small doses, usually found in fruits and vegetables, have a bio-positive effect while the larger doses help the squamous cell carcinoma by their bio-negative role.

The world famous Misasa hot springs that are known for their disease curing effects emanate radon waves in very small doses—the radium decay products. Radon, in small doses, found around the Misasa springs, produced by the hot water fumes coming out of the spring waters there, stimulates the body's immune system. Since radon cannot penetrate human skin, the fumes here are breathed in by the tourists and patients who go there. Radon, when it enters the human body through the lungs, works efficiently as an anti-oxidant through the super-oxide desmutase system. The Mesasa springs are famous for curing autoimmune diseases like rheumatoid arthritis.

In an earlier article I had shown how eating fruits and vegetables, unlike daily intake of multivitamins, is health promoting. One could understand the scientific rationale behind this if one realizes the hormetic effect of all the vitamins, both water soluble and fat soluble ones. Modern medical therapeutics could learn a lesson or two from the hormetic concept. The human body responds in a non-linear fashion in any situation. Linear systems do not work in the human body. We have to rethink our dose-response curves in pharmacology. Let me remind the reader that well over 150,000 people die every year in the US alone due to unforeseen drug side effects. Understanding hormesis could reduce this burden significantly.

The one man who has worked very hard on this hormetic concept is Professor Edward Calabrese of the University of Massachusetts. This concept would take away the sail from many groups fighting against environmental pollution. Whereas it is true that heavily polluted environment is bad for human health some degree of pollution is inevitable in the modern day world. Extremism in any field has harmful effects on humanity. If we want one hundred per cent pollution free environment, we should be prepared to go back to the Stone Age. Even there people did have background radiation hazards that kept them alive, I suppose. Nature knows best. "What an ingenious medley is Nature's: if our faces were not alike, we could not tell man from beast: if they were not unlike we could not tell man from man," wrote Michel de Montaigne.

Even the stones in the Stone Age did emanate small doses of radon with the sun shining on them. This might have prolonged human life span then! Similarly, most chemical poisons, in very small doses, work as anti-oxidants, as shown above. I must hasten to add that this knowledge should not mislead the greedy multinational companies to pollute the globe heavily with their greed for profits and their proclivity for comfort. It is only when man poisons the last river, cuts the last tree, and chemically loads the last bit of earth would he realize that money cannot be eaten to survive. Moderation in everything makes life happier. Small IS beautiful as Schumacher had shown. Fanaticism leads to terrorism. Many times it is the intellectual terrorism that is more dangerous than the weapons of mass destruction kind of terrorism, like the one reported above about the (in) famous Linus Pauling.

It is the scientific performance rather than the scientific conception that tends to bewilder the lay public.
—Peter Medawar, in *The Limits of Science,* 1986

Afterword

DEEP DOWN MODERN MEDICAL SCIENCE IS VERY SHALLOW

"Silence is the greatest enemy of social good" wrote Amartya Sen, the Nobel Laureate economist, in his latest book *Argumentative India*. I couldn't agree more. Modern medicine, with its misguided scientific base, has been counterproductive in its effect on society, to put it mildly. Although there have been occasional voices here and there expressing their concerns, I have not found any one daring to challenge the establishment. My half-a-Century's experience (from the time I joined the medical school in 1956) has made me feel that we are trying to keep the medical students in the dark about the truth. Like in other fields of learning and teaching we never let our students *think* for themselves! Despite the fact that students today have easy access to original research unlike in our student days, most of the inconvenient data is kept under the wraps by the vested interests.

I, therefore, decided that it was time to "talk of many things, cabbages and kings," as the Walrus said, in this field in no uncertain terms to make the medical profession aware of the real truth behind what we are doing and what is expected of us by society. While doctors are trained to keep the health of the public, we do not let doctors in training to know what that is all about. Health preservation (keeping the well healthy) is not stressed in the curriculum at all. Most, if not all, doctors are under the impression that the quick-fix interventions are the be-all and end-all of a doctor's duty. The divine interventionists and their masters in the industry are projected as the saviours of mankind. While the real truth is that overinvestigations and unnecessary interventions had resulted in thousands of unnecessary deaths even in the US: the medical care in the US being the worst among the 14 developed countries studied. That exactly is the compelling reason to write this book.

The encouragement that I received from Prof Rustom Roy, the father of nanotechnology, has been my motivation. I hope that this book will open the eyes of the future generations of doctors to appreciate the real pleasures of doctoring. I have tried to keep them informed of the correct scientific basis of modern medicine, in addition. Extensive references would enable an interested student to go deep into the roots of the problem, if needed.

A few outsiders had tried in the past to give the lay readers a peep hole view of the inner working of the medical establishment with all its inherent dangers. The leading figures have been Norman Cousins, Ivan Illich and Thomas McKevon; but that has been only the tip of the iceberg. An insider has better access to the real truths and will be able to authoritatively write on it. There have been few attempts lately by Marcia Angell, Barbra Starfield and John Abramson, but they touched on bits and pieces only. I would not like to say that I have found **the** truth, but would only say that I have found **a** truth. Science is change and change is life. Student is advised to keep in touch with the fast growing information overload in the field of medical literature. Although most of it is only *noise,* an occasional *signal* should never be missed. A committed teacher could play a vital role in this area as a facilitator.

A word of caution here though. Never take anything lying down. Most of what comes out in medical literature is not the truth. Medical literature is doctored, tutored, and "sexed up" by the powers-that-be before being allowed to be published. Knowledge dwells in heads replete with thoughts of other men, but wisdom dwells in heads attentive to their own. Be a thinker and think about all the myths that I have tried to demolish in this book. If you could improve upon what I have written here my goal in writing this book will have been achieved. *My aim is to make every doctor a learner*. Let us not let medical science stagnate for Centuries as it did in the past. One example is in order here. It was in the year 127 AD that Galen, the venerated teacher, wrote that blood circulated mainly from the liver. For 1400 odd years every medical teacher and researcher replicated that (in) "famous truth." It took the courage of William Harvey in 1628 AD to write *de Motu Cordis* and show that blood circulated from the heart. We, in India knew all about the functions of the heart for thousands of years. Ayurveda had discussed this accurately thousands of years ago. That is the beauty of Indian wisdom.

I also deem it my duty to let the students know that this book and its contents should not be reproduced in the examination papers as the conventional thinking examiners might not approve of it. When one qualifies, one has to unlearn all that one had learnt in the medical school to relearn the real life medicine. This book is hoped to help that difficult process of relearning. Later on this book might help one to get answers to knotty problems in daily life. I only hope that my efforts do not go in vain. Send us your suggestions for improvement of the future editions.

He makes no friends who never made a foe.
—Alfred, Lord Tennyson